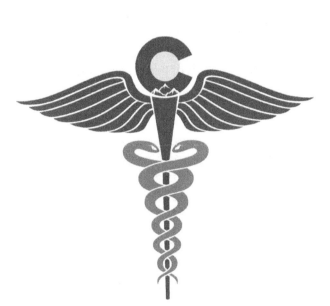

Colorado Medical Solutions

Foreword

By: Dr. Eric Akin MD Neurosurgeon

In the timeless pursuit of health and well-being, humanity has long grappled with a singular, pervasive challenge – the struggle to maintain a healthy weight. This relentless battle against the bulge has touched every corner of the globe, transcending age, gender, and culture. It is, without a doubt, the biggest problem plaguing our species. Yet, within the heart of this enigmatic struggle lies the key to our longevity, vitality, and the pursuit of a flourishing life

"Fast, Feast, & Flourish" by Dr. Dean Jones is a beacon of hope for those navigating this perplexing journey. This book delves deep into the very heart of the issue and provides an evidence-based roadmap to sustainable weight loss, empowering you to take control of your metabolic destiny

In a world awash with fad diets, unfulfilled promises, and conflicting advice, "Fast, Feast, & Flourish" swiftly gets to the point. Dr. Jones recognizes the urgency of the problem and aims to equip you with practical tools for success from the outset. This book is not a compendium of quick fixes or miracle cures, but a carefully crafted guide based on solid scientific research

One of the book's most compelling features is its ability to offer a bird's-eye view of the formidable obstacles that have stymied our efforts to address the weight gain crisis. Through the FLOA Protocol, Dr. Jones sheds light on the intricate web of metabolic processes that govern our bodies. By understanding these mechanisms, you can make informed choices, unshackling yourself from the relentless cycle of weight gain and loss

Additionally, "Fast, Feast, & Flourish" pulls back the curtain on the weight loss industry, revealing the shortfalls that have left countless individuals feeling disheartened and defeated. Dr. Jones calls for a paradigm shift, advocating for an approach that focuses on sustainable health rather than quick fixes that ultimately lead to disappointment

In a world where misinformation abounds, this book serves as a lifeline to those who yearn for lasting change. Dr. Dean Jones, a recognized authority in the field, has poured his expertise, passion, and dedication into these pages. "Fast, Feast, & Flourish" will challenge the way you perceive weight management, guiding you toward a healthier, happier, and more fulfilling life

It is our hope that the knowledge contained within these chapters will empower you to take control of your metabolic destiny, conquer the challenge of weight maintenance, and ultimately, enable you to flourish.

Praise

"Fast, Feast, & Flourish" is a comprehensive guide that provides a fresh perspective on weight loss and maintenance. As an RN with a deep understanding of metabolic health, I appreciate the book's scientific approach to weight management, particularly its focus on insulin sensitivity and the role of GLP-1 medications and peptides. The author, Dr. Dean Jones, shares his personal weight loss journey, which adds a relatable and motivational aspect to the book. His FLOA protocol is not only backed by science but also broken down into easy-to-follow steps, making it accessible to anyone. I particularly value Dr. Jones' approach to using medications as a temporary aid rather than a long-term solution. This book will undoubtedly serve as a valuable resource for healthcare professionals and individuals seeking sustainable weight loss solutions."
Yvette Oxford RN

"Fast, Feast, & Flourish" is a compelling read that offers a fresh perspective on weight management. As a chiropractor with over 20 years of experience, I found the book's holistic approach to weight loss and maintenance particularly enlightening. The author's emphasis on the FLOA protocol, a structured fasting program, challenges conventional calorie-based weight loss methods that often lead to failure. The book also delves into the financial and research biases that can skew our understanding of effective weight loss strategies, providing a critical lens through which to view existing research. The author's personal journey with weight loss adds a layer of authenticity and relatability to the narrative. This book is a valuable resource for anyone in the health field, offering insights that can enhance patient care and outcomes in weight management."

Dr Dan Alexander

"The FLOA system combines the ancient and the modern to create an amalgam that cuts to the core of fat burning for healthy sustained weight loss. A revolutionary force to transform your life, your health and your happiness. Dr. Jones has created a juggernaut system to unlock the issues of modern day obesity and other metabolic diseases based on his personal journey and clinical experience that has helped thousands of patients live healthier lives. As a physician of 30 years who left the disease care system to help people reverse disease by going to the root cause, Dr. Jones also goes to the root cause of obesity. Bravo"

Roberto Tostado M.D- Author of WTF is wrong with our health? A Rebel physician's manifesto for reversing disease and increase smiles

"Fast, Feast, & Flourish" by Dr. Dean Jones and Jonathan Keith is a comprehensive guide that offers a unique and scientifically backed approach to weight loss and maintenance. As a doctorate of acupuncture and functional medicine specialist, I appreciate the book's holistic approach to weight management. The authors introduce the FLOA Protocol, a method that combines the use of GLP-1 medications and peptides with strategic fasting, allowing individuals to wean off medications while maintaining their weight loss. The book is not just about the science of weight loss, but also about the personal journey of Dr. Jones, who shares his own experiences with weight loss, providing a relatable and motivational narrative for readers. The FLOA protocol is presented in a step-by-step manner, making it easy to follow. The authors' approach to using medications when necessary, but not as a long-term solution, aligns with the principles of functional medicine. This

book is a valuable resource for anyone seeking a sustainable and holistic approach to weight loss."
Dan Kellams DACM, L.Ac

"FAST, FEAST, & FLOURISH by Dr. Dean Jones and Jonathan Keith is an excellent guide to losing weight and keeping it off.

As a Family Practice physician for 35 years, I have encouraged thousands of overweight patients to eat correctly. I used as my motto to losing weight, "How goes my weight, so goes my health." This is not true in all cases, but it emphasizes how important maintaining a healthy weight is. I also tried to encourage weight loss without medications, but instead to change eating habits and to exercise. This book brilliantly adds another important element, prolonged fasting. Dr. Jones' "Prolonged Fasting Schedule" may be exactly what many need to finally lose weight and keep it off. I have looked at his recommendations and can wholeheartedly recommend each carefully planned step as outlined in his book."
Dr. Dan Hale

"This book is fantastic at explaining how fasting can remain part of one's lifestyle in order to keep one "insulin sensitive". Dr. Jones shows vulnerability by telling his story, which allows readers to relate and gives them a sense of motivation. The FLOA protocol is backed by science, which I can appreciate, but it's also sustainable. The method is broken down into steps that make it easy for anyone to follow. I love Dr. Jones' approach to using medications when applicable, but not as a long-term fix. I will use this book as revenge when helping my own clients achieve metabolic health through fasting, fiber, and tools such as the Feel Great System."
Shannon Davis, RD, LD

Table of Contents

The Essential Reasons
Why You Should Read This Book

It all started with going through my weight loss journey of over 100lbs when I was 16 years old. I lost the weight but struggled to keep it off for over a decade. I discovered how fasting for longer periods of time was the answer for me. Intermittent fasting was a good start, but the magic happened when I progressed into doing longer rounds of fasting. After becoming a doctor of Chiropractic, I started working with patients to help them with their functional health. For over the last decade, I've taken many of them through a journey from short to prolonged fasting programs. What I have been able to see first-hand over the years through clinical observation and blood chemistry analysis has been nothing short of miraculous. The flashy new weight loss medications, Semaglutide and Tirzepatide are changing the obesity market as we know it. Unfortunately, they require lifelong adherence; like many other medications do. I have a solution for this. Everything has led me to this point. I have created a scientifically backed solution that will not only make it much easier for you to lose weight compared to what you have tried in the past, but more importantly, it will set you up for success in maintaining the weight loss for the rest of your life. This is my promise to you.

This is a manageable guide to weight loss. A quick guide to understanding what has been our secret at Colorado Medical Solutions to deliver this wildly successful program. Countless lives have improved by losing weight this way. Many patients have reported that for the first time, they have something tangible they can follow. That gives them confidence in their ability to lose weight and **maintain it afterward**. It is very observable that obesity is getting much worse. All efforts to help have failed miserably. **The FLOA™ (pronounced "Flow") Protocol has allowed us to**

1

combine the best practices of two completely parallel worlds: clinical perspective combined with a holistic approach incorporating ancestral wisdom and increasing one thing: your PLAY span.

Scan here to see FLOA Weight Loss TESTIMONIALS!

Weight loss is a highly complex subject, so many people struggle with it. Just look at the obesity rate in America; it continues to climb. A new study in the *Lancet Medical Journal* found that for the first time in history, obese people now outnumber underweight people! In 2014, 641 million people were obese, compared to 175 million in 1975. By 2025, an estimated 20% of the global population and about ½ of Americans will be obese! People require help with weight loss. But it necessitates a correct understanding of the real problem driving obesity: Insulin. Without this understanding first and building solutions around it; we're just spinning our wheels. The other concern is that weight loss programs aren't easy enough for people to implement in their stress-filled lives. Unfortunately, the programs that are easy enough to implement are gimmicky and unhealthy. Easy, sustainable, and healthy weight loss programs are not something I have seen much of. Look at this scary statistic, "Only about 20% of Americans who lose weight can keep it off long term, (research) has found."(187) Clearly, what's on the market in terms of weight loss does an inferior job at setting people up for success with maintaining the weight loss

The government's attempt to wage war on obesity has failed over and over. Hundreds of millions of dollars are spent on campaigns to combat obesity, while it only gets worse at alarming rates. Despite the continual failure; they continue to promote the same ideology of eating small meals throughout the day and a diet rich in carbs. They say it's all about calories. We just need to eat less and move more. I believe Einstein said insanity is defined as "running the same experiment over and over and expecting a different result." Maybe they know it isn't working and prefer it that way? Another time and book for my feelings on all that!

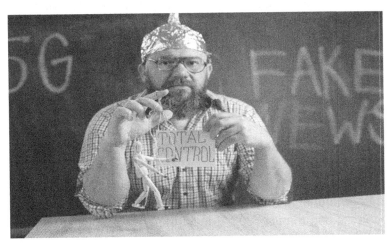

The trend in the industry recently has been all about the medication **SEMAGLUTIDE**. This medication is going viral because of its ability to suppress appetite dramatically. Many celebrities are showcasing their dramatic changes. The running joke among the wealthy has been, "who's not on Semaglutide, raise your hand." The problem with only artificially suppressing appetite to drop weight is the high likelihood that they will regain it. A recent randomized controlled trial concluded that:

One year after withdrawal of once-weekly subcutaneous semaglutide 2.4 mg and lifestyle intervention, participants regained two-thirds of their prior weight loss, with similar changes in cardio metabolic variables. Findings confirm the chronicity of obesity and suggest ongoing treatment is required to maintain improvements in weight and health. (186)

That is with some sort of lifestyle intervention that was paired with the medication! Think about it for a minute. We already had a massive issue with people's ability to keep off the weight after they lost it. What would adding a powerful appetite suppressant do? It allows more people who don't have the proper mindset and structure to lose weight in a way that fosters maintenance to now suddenly lose weight. What does this mean for their ability to keep it off afterward?

There are three ways to look at this. There are millions of people who picked this up from a med spa or a clinic that is not properly guiding them. Many people are experiencing first hand just how dramatic the rebound of weight is after stopping the medication. The 2nd way is under an educated obesity specialist who goes off the data and understands that obesity is a disease and therefore requires lifelong medication. At least they are practicing ethically within the framework they understand and are experienced in. Finally, there is our way. We utilize these medications to help initially reprogram your relationship with food. A lot of you are too inflamed and insulin resistant to break through the initial food chatter otherwise. With this new sense of self-control, we utilize the FLOA protocol, which aggressively handles the underlying mechanism driving the disease to begin with. Then, we can successfully wean you off the medications. We have helped thousands do so. (We also work with people who don't want to start with the medications).

I am a massive fan of these new medications that we call GLP-1s. They give us the opportunity to reprogram our brains regarding our relationship with food. BAM...... the food chatter is gone. That never-ending sense of hunger is severely dampened. With this effect, something magical can happen afterward. Despite the study's grim look, our patients see something very different. The "lifestyle" approach that we take is something entirely different from something you have ever seen before. You may be familiar with fasting and even be familiar with prolonged fasting. But you are unfamiliar with the FLOA protocol unless you have already worked with us or know someone who has. 😃 This has been my life's work creating this wildly successful approach.

I'm attempting to give you an easy-to-do weight loss and maintenance strategy to provide you with DRAMATIC RESULTS. Something that you will find easy to navigate around in a busy life: I promise.

I will discuss why it's currently so difficult to win the battle of obesity and healthy weight management. Then, I dive into the science behind the problem and the science of the solutions. Then we end with the mechanics of our program

If you desire to watch my webinar series before reading this book, scan the QR code below. Take some time to watch the webinars.

They will give you an overall summary and are broken up into three parts.

Before you start reading – start the challenge

I want you to see just how easy it is to start fasting. If you have never done this before, let's start by eating your first meal one hour later than what you are used to. This goes for your 1st meal or any form of calories. Whatever time that is, let's push that by a single hour and every 3 days to a week when you feel that is easier, go ahead and push that one more hour. Why should you do this?

1. It will improve your confidence that you were able to start fasting.
2. It will begin to affect your body positively in ways that will start to promote weight loss.
3. Your microbiome will begin to heal and improve itself, as well as your health.
4. You will likely start to sleep better.
5. Your body will get into deeper stages of healing.
6. You may start to feel better overall.

Truthfully, I can go on and on and I will throughout this book. But these are some of the wonderful things that happen to your body when you begin to incorporate this amazing lifestyle strategy into your daily regime. And it's free-99 ☺

If you already have experience fasting, then, begin to push wherever it is that you are at. If you are already successfully doing a daily 8-hour eating window, you can push that to 7 or 6. Or you can start one 24 hours per week. There are no failures here. Every time you set out to challenge yourself and increase the fasting window more than the prior time is a win in my book. Enjoy the satisfaction of knowing that you are not only challenging yourself, but literally, you will live longer because of it!

Medical Disclaimers

This book is intended to provide general information about medical weight loss, fasting, peptides, and holistic medicine. The author, a Doctor of Chiropractic, is not a medical doctor and does not hold a degree in medicine. The content in this book is based on the author's personal experiences, opinions, and research

The information provided in this book is for informational and educational purposes only and should not be considered as a substitute for professional medical advice, diagnosis, or treatment. Always consult a qualified healthcare professional before making any decisions or changes to your health regimen, especially if you have a pre-existing medical condition

The author and publisher of this book make no representations or warranties, express or implied, regarding the accuracy, reliability, or completeness of the content provided. They disclaim any liability for any errors, omissions, or inaccuracies in the information provided. The author and publisher are not responsible for any adverse effects or consequences resulting from the use or misuse of any information, suggestions, or procedures described in this book

In no event shall the author or publisher be liable for any direct, indirect, incidental, special, consequential, or punitive damages arising out of or in connection with the use of this book. By reading and using the information in this book, you agree to assume full responsibility for your health and well-being and release the author and publisher from any liability related to the content of this book

If you have any concerns or questions about your health, consult a qualified healthcare professional before making any changes to your health regimen. Do not disregard professional medical advice or delay seeking it because of something you have read in this book.

IMPORTANT! All information presented in this book is intended for informational purposes only and not for the purpose of rendering medical advice. Statements made in this book have not been evaluated by the Food and Drug Administration. The information contained herein is not intended to diagnose, treat, cure or prevent any disease.

Who am I?

Colorado Medical Solutions Mission Statement – Thoroughly and effectively treated patients who are happy and refer others because we utilize the most cutting-edge healthcare services that aim to reduce prescriptions, prevent surgeries when possible,and restore optimal health Dr. Dean Jones, DC

My name is Dr. Dean Jones, DC, a Chiropractic Physician. I am the founder and owner of Colorado Medical Solutions in Denver and Colorado Springs. Our medically integrated practices specialize in anti-aging services, with a big emphasis on Weight Loss and bio-identical Hormone Therapy. My background is in Functional Health and weight loss with our patients. Functional Health is what I consider "real" healthcare.

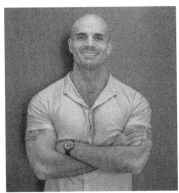

This approach allows us to deeply dive into our patient's health, uncover many disease processes before they progress, and help reverse them through lifestyle management that usually consists of supplements, nutrition, exercise, and stress management. Over the years of doing this, I realized only the wealthy can afford real functional health, so I started developing protocols in our clinic that bring over the "flavor of functional health" but are much more reasonably priced. Colorado Medical Solutions continues to grow by helping people get off prescription drugs, preventing surgeries when possible, and restoring optimal health. It's incredible what practitioners unravel when they aren't bound by "what the insurance companies will cover."

My biggest passion in life, hands down, is helping them with their weight loss. Nothing else in this world brings me more joy. My personal experience with being overweight in the past and the years I struggled to maintain it afterward gave me the ability to really understand where people are coming from. To see what they are dealing with while on their journey to a better version of themselves. I love the group format of group coaching that we do for our patients and being able to inspire others through their weight loss struggles.

I grew up as a normal child at a normal weight, but you could see the excess pounds slowly starting to creep in by the age of six to eight. As I grew older, it continued to get worse. I find this to be a tough age to be overweight, as it's more difficult for a child to be aware of the implications of being overweight. By the time I made it to the 5th grade, I began to become aware that I was overweight. Or like the other kids enjoined pointing out to me all the time: "fat." Recent empirical evidence suggests there are multiple levels of awareness, and the stage at which a child becomes aware of their body and how it compares to others begins in adolescence but continues to develop into adulthood.(2) For me, it was that 9-12 age range where I started introverting hard. It just kept getting worse year by year. I kept gaining more and more weight, and I kept feeling worse and worse about myself. This was the turning point in my life where I began to go down a bad path. Up to this point, I would describe my life as "awesome!" I had friends, and we hung out and played video games and did what most kids did at that point in their lives. I look back and see how I made myself an easy target for bullies. I really let it affect me for whatever reason. I had never dealt with that before. I really struggled to make new friends from that point on. Furthermore, I chose to use food as my fix. I would eat more frequently and look for that junk food high that would make me feel better. The irony in all this was that I had healthy parents who noticed that I was gaining a lot of weight. My mom was overweight as a child but lost weight, got healthy and maintained it for the rest of her life. They did their best to feed me healthy food and encouraged more exercise, but it didn't help. I managed to sneak in the junk food one way or another, and I avoided social settings. The crazy thing though was I never made the real connection that it all stemmed from my weight. Even after starting high school, I still didn't make any connections between my feelings about myself and my excess weight

High school was miserable for me. I was picked on and bullied more than others. I had no confidence in who I was as a young man. Furthermore, I continued in a downward spiral of eating junk food and feeling bad about myself. At this point, my parents had less control over what I ate, as I bought my food at school for lunch. I would eat pizza, hamburgers, tacos, burritos, chips, soda, cookies, and just about any delicious treat I could get my hands on. High school was a real struggle for me just to survive. I always wondered why life was the way it was for me. Around my early junior year of high school, I finally made the connection that it had to do with my weight. For whatever reason, I still failed to decide to do something about it. Looking back, it makes sense. I was so depressed about who I was and the life I was living. I was barely surviving! Research shows that food has a massive impact on mental health. (3) I'll never forget the day when I was 16 years old in a 24-hour fitness locker room. I went to the gym occasionally, believe it or not. But I certainly was not actively trying to lose weight, as I had not decided yet to do so. I stepped on the scale that day, and it exceeded 300 pounds. I cannot begin to describe the feelings I experienced seeing my weight pass the BIG 300. Keep in mind, I was a non-muscular kid. We're not talking about a big, strong football lineman who was 300lbs. We are talking 300 lbs of pure fat! I lost my ability to complete a single push-up when I weighed around 260lbs. On this day, though, it was different. I stared at the scale. I re-weighed myself a few times, thinking it could be some error. No errors. A rush of feelings came over me, but the biggest one was FEAR. I started realizing that this weight gain was getting to a point where "real" health complications were around the corner. The doctors had already told my parents and me that changes needed to be made ASAP! My cholesterol, triglycerides (the primary type of fat in our body), and hemoglobin A1c (measure of average blood sugar levels and indicator of diabetes) were all very high for my age. None of these things seemed to scare me beforehand. But on this day, I was full of fear at the gym. The rest of the day, all I did was think about the path that I was on. After a few hours of panicking, I then rose to a point of anger. Within a day of being angry, I felt motivated to take action. I was pissed, but I felt more in control. I had risen above the apathetic tone that I was letting myself live in. I told myself, "I can do this! I can lose this weight and change my life!" It's incredible how something can trigger and improve someone's confidence by changing their viewpoint to make it more optimistic. It was a survival-driven response that turned into my operating basis. This was the turning point for me in my life

After that day, I began researching everything I could get my hands on that had to do with weight loss. The consensus was obvious: I needed to eat healthier, eat less food, lift weights, and do cardio. So, that's what I did. Over the next year, I managed to lose 100 pounds and transform my life for the better. By the time I reached the age of 18 years old, I had become a personal trainer for 24-hour fitness clubs, as I wanted to help inspire others struggling with their weight issues. I became a master trainer within a year, and received three different personal training certifications. The consensus of my education on weight loss at that time was the same, really; eat less and burn more. I did start to observe patterns in my clients. There was a lot of rebound weight gain. I didn't think much more of it, as it was something that I also personally dealt with. My attitude was simply, "mind over matter." I was going to college and fulfilling my prerequisites for a health profession. At the time, I knew I wanted to be a doctor. However, I was unsure about the specialty. My career in the gym became an essential step in my life. I ended up becoming the Training General Manager for LA

Fitness gyms at the age of 19. I was passionate about helping my trainers get the best results with their clients. From that position, I more clearly saw the issue within their clients after losing weight. But nothing came from that observation yet

A few years later, an annoying wrist injury led me to Chiropractic and holistic health. I fractured my wrist in a bad fall, and it failed to heal properly. Two negative MRIs and four months of time passed after the injury, only to be told by two orthopedic surgeons, "Sometimes it just takes time." I knew something was wrong. A member at my gym overheard me talking about my injury and recommended a Chiropractor; I had no clue they could help with injuries outside the spine. Desperately, I went to see the Chiropractor. After just two treatments, I was able to use my wrist again. It took me only one month of seeing this Chiropractor before I discovered what I wanted to do. I still wanted to be a doctor, but I wanted to focus on helping people in a healthcare setting which was more holistic in nature. I returned to school to finish my undergrad requirements. I headed to *Southern California University of Health Sciences* for my Doctorate of Chiropractic. Working alongside like-minded medical practitioners allowed me to deliver the best holistic healthcare I could. In doing so, I learned while Chiropractic can be life changing, it is only one component of several to achieve *optimal health*. Quickly in my career, I medically integrated my clinics. For the last decade, I have been working alongside medical practitioners to provide the most cutting-edge healthcare services that aim to reduce prescriptions, prevent surgeries when possible and restore optimal health!

So, I dropped 100 lbs and dramatically changed my life at 16. I mean dramatically! I finally began to accept myself and develop socially, something I refrained from in the past. I'm sure most readers here are way past this point, and more likely gained their weight in adulthood. I'm just sharing my history with you all to show you why I have a passion for all this. . Unfortunately, I failed to maintain a healthy weight. Every year I struggled again and had to re-lose 30-50 lbs come February/March. This pattern continued until my mid-20s. I never let myself regain all my weight and get back to 300lbs, but my weight did fluctuate from 210 to 260. The thought of summer coming up always fueled me to get back into shape. As I grew older, I began to see this bad habit of mine and tried my best to not regain so much weight every fall and winter. Better discipline and understanding of human physiology and various tricks and tips helped for sure. However, my biggest breakthrough was my exposure to intermittent fasting. I was 22 years old when I started reading about it, and I swear I thought it was a crazy idea. Years of eating small meals 5 to 6 times a day had me "drinking the proverbial kool-aid." Additionally, most bodybuilders I knew were not doing any sort of fasting during their cutting phases, let alone at all. Cutting is when they focus their attention on dropping body fat while maintaining muscle mass. I eventually gave it a shot. Within a year my annual fluctuation of weight was 50% improved. Wow! This fasting thing really blew my mind. It clashed with so much information that I understood to be true. I was pretty attuned with my body by that point. I understood what the shift in my calories and exercise could do in either direction, and how much effort it took me to drop fat. But it seemed as if there was some other driving force behind the improvements I experienced when I started fasting. Yes, fasting provides some calorie restriction, no doubt. However, this was entirely unique. It was like I didn't have to try as hard to drop fat, and I didn't seem to put on the fat so easily as before.

Fast-forward into my early years of practice in my late 20s. By this point, I would say I achieved the ability to maintain a level of body fat that I was happy with, but it still required great effort. More effort than I thought it should. I was now balancing the effort it took for me to be as lean as I wanted to with the effort I more importantly needed for the rest of my life! I really think this is part of the dilemma that people experience

Is this extra weight a big enough problem for me to justify the extra amount of effort and sacrifice it will take to accomplish losing it now?

Sadly for many, it's just not. It's unfortunate because these people will eventually face health consequences due to extra weight that continues to creep in. It's easy to ignore it in your 20s, 30s and 40s. But eventually, you are hit with reality. Now you are pre-diabetic, have high cholesterol and feel like crap. Or worse, now you are obese. How did this happen? You recall being fit and healthy with little attention to it, and now this?! Now all of a sudden, the concern is big enough, and now you are scrambling to do something about it. Anyhow, end of rant and back to my story. So I was explaining that I went through times when, if I chose to do so, I could stay in shape. If I could just manage to keep it high enough on my priority list, there would have been no issue. Generally, I decided that the other areas of my life, such as opening up my practices, were far more important to me.

Eventually, I was exposed to prolonged fasting, about ten years ago. This is where the real magic set in. Once I became proficient at prolonged fasting, it was now "easy" to stay in shape. It was also easier for me to get real lean when I wanted to do all that. I finally felt normal regarding the amount of effort it took to stay at a healthy athletic body fat percentage. I became obsessed with prolonged fasting. I started to study every book, journal, podcasts, and even YouTube resource I could find. You name it, I studied it. I soon learned how much more prolonged fasting does for improving health. At this time, intermittent fasting was still the new kid on the block, let alone prolonged fasting. Working with patients in the functional space, I started incorporating prolonged fasting into their health optimization programs. I can't tell you how many patients thought I was nuts, but would trust me and take my advice. I was blown away by the outcomes I would see. The blood and stool analysis tests were powerful objective indicators that something powerful was happening. We will dive into the excellent benefits of fasting and how much better prolonged fasting is for you than just the more popularized intermittent fasting later on.

However, structure was missing in the world of prolonged fasting. This led me to create the FLOA protocol, which I believe to be the world's most aggressive approach towards extended fasting. I was fortunate enough to see firsthand how safe and effective prolonged fasting is for health and longevity, but, more importantly, that it's the most powerful tool for weight management. So, I created this protocol to give structure where the structure was needed in the hopes of helping to slow down this obesity epidemic we find ourselves in. I have coached thousands of people to implement this protocol successfully and helped them obtain healthy weight management for the first time.

This book is about implementing a successful prolonged fasting schedule so that you can become proficient and utilize it after that to stay in shape with much more "ease" than ever before. I believe this to be the missing piece that would allow many more people to drop weight and, more importantly, keep it off for the rest of their lives.

Jonathan Keith – Clinics Director

Contributing Writer

Oh, man, where to start?

Close your eyes and imagine the awkward, skinny kid with few friends and many neurotic quirks. That was me – curious, petite, and a late bloomer. But fast-forward to my time as an undergraduate at CSUF, where I met Dr. Jones (I didn't call him that at the time), the Fitness Director for LA Fitness. He took me under his wing, and I quickly realized that anything related to the human body and how it could be kept in top form, naturally, just sat in my brain and rested

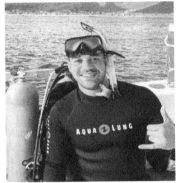

I was hooked. Over the next decade, I climbed the ranks of the fitness industry, learning from and being mentored by some of the best-and-brightest individuals I have ever encountered. And now, as the Director and Integrative Health Expert for Colorado Medical Solutions, I've been given the opportunity of a lifetime: to help build an empire to help prevent surgeries, reduce medications, and restore optimal health

As someone who has been in the health field for over 15 years, I have come to find a true passion for increasing the "play span" of as many individuals as possible. The quality of life is just as important as the number of days spent on this earth. Through my focus on functional health integration, rehab, nutrition, and biomechanics, I've found that the only way to help people is not

17

through a cookie-cutter or one-size-fits-all technique but rather a constant individualized approach that is constantly evolving

I've particularly excelled in health optimization and coaching using lab results to help patients to understand how to eat better and take the right supplements to avoid taking the medications their doctors normally prescribe, such as statins, which can be harmful. It's incredibly rewarding to see patients improve their health and avoid unnecessary medications by making simple lifestyle changes

Over the years, the number of patients who have thanked us for getting them off their drugs or improving their quality of life has been overwhelming. It's a testament to the power of functional health and the importance of personalized care

Of course, the health, and wellness field is constantly evolving, and my approach has changed along with it. I used to sit in a chair facing my clients and spout things like "Eat breakfast like a king, lunch like a prince, and dinner like a peasant" and "Don't consume anything at bedtime because your body will go into hibernation mode!" But now, we know the tremendous health benefits of prolonged fasting leading to autophagy, and how the "eat all day" concept has led to a spike in insulin resistance

Despite these changes, my biggest joy professionally remains hearing the success stories of people who have legitimately had their lives changed for the better. The look on someone's face when you cut their triglycerides in half in six weeks with nothing but supplemental intervention and minor lifestyle changes is enough to keep me going every single day

It's frustrating that so many people out there are making true attempts to control their health, only to be met by clouds of misinformation with the pure intent of nothing but profit. That's why

I'm so passionate about what I do – because I know that by focusing on functional health and personalized care, we can make a real difference in people's lives.

The Quick Protocol

I know a large swath of you will want to start immediately. So here's the protocol boiled down to the most basic form possible.

1. Weekly weigh-ins
    a. It's important to stay as consistent as possible with your weekly weigh-ins. If it's Tuesday morning, then do your best to keep it every Tuesday morning. This allows you to alter course when necessary. The biggest benefit is the ability to catch a plateau as it's happening and fix it and get back on course.
    b. You can record in your app of choice, or use the notes app on your phone.
    c. This is your gauge to ensure you are losing weight and not slowing down your metabolism. You should lose 0.5-1.5% of your body weight per week once you hit the FLOA stage, as described below. Noting trends of decreasing losses or no loss are indications that you plateaued. See below on how to address this.
    d. Plan now, ahead of time, what days you think your weekly long fast will be, so you can start weight tracking now on that day for consistencies' sake. You **DO NOT** want to weigh yourself 12 hours or later into your fast, as you will drop a lot of water weight, and it makes the results harder to interpret.

    e. For example, if you eat dinner Monday evening and start the fast afterward, your weekly weigh-in should be Monday or Tuesday AM.

    f. This should also be the same time as your weekly Semaglutide/Tirzepatide shot if you intend to use it, as the appetite-suppressing effects could wear off after a few days into each 7-day cycle.

2. Diet

    a. I prefer Mediterranean and/or Paleo. If you have any sort of autoimmune disease, then you should be following a more strict anti-inflammation diet. I want an unrestricted diet for you as much as possible, as I believe that is one of the keys to long-term sustainable weight loss. Google and ChatGPT have more than enough information for you to find ideas of how to eat and what to eat within these categories. If you are not losing weight, then you can start to restrict your diet more, focusing on cutting out more inflammatory foods. The strictest diets you will find are your autoimmune diets. See appendix for some examples.

    b. Start a Keto version of the above. I know Keto is not sustainable for most people long term, so I'm only asking you to do it for a few months. There is a better response initially to the FLOA if you make it happen for the first month until you hit the weekly 48-hour fast stage. Go as low-carb/keto as you can! Do not stress about hitting the 0–20 grams of net carbs (carb) required to actually hit ketosis, but if you can, then great.

    c. Adhere to the 90/10 rule. You know what junk food is. But allow me to spell it out for you:

        i. Highly processed foods

      ii.   Vegetable and seed oils

     iii.   Trans Fats

     iv.   Fried foods

      v.   High-sugar foods

     vi.   High insulin-producing foods.

          1.   There are foods that are low in sugar but, despite the fact, still produce a high insulin response. The insulin index shows you the rating of how much insulin particular foods produce. Sneaky food examples to avoid in the beginning are: Low-fat dairy products, beans, and lean fish.

  d. All these bad foods fall into the 10%. I could tell you to avoid them, but could you really sustain that for the rest of your life? The FLOA is so powerful that most people will do just fine to keep them at 10% or less.

      i.   NOTE – Some severe insulin resistant and chronically inflamed cases will require 100% adherence through the first few months to heal the damage that is present.

  e. Ensure adequate protein. About 1 gram of protein per pound of what you want to weigh is a good, easy metric to follow.

3. Assessing the Weight Loss Plateau

  a. We need to assess if you are in a current Weight Loss Plateau before starting any more weight loss. This is a state where your metabolism has slowed down. You NEVER should start working towards weight loss from this point, as you will likely slow down your metabolism even more. This is crucial for long-term success. The following are examples of a plateau:

i.   You tried to lose weight, and it was working, and now it stopped.

ii.   If you have been on a GLP1 medication for a month or more, then you are likely in some plateau. Even if weight loss is still happening upon starting this program.

iii.   You were losing weight, and it stalled, and you have been stuck there for however long. Since then, exercising the same amount of time and/or eating the same amount, usually out of fear of regaining weight.

iv.   You have been in a caloric deficit. Figure out how many calories you have been averaging. And then compare it to this estimator. https://tdeecalculator.net/

v.   You are dealing with lower energy, brain fog, constipation, hair loss, body aches , intolerance to cold, and you recall that it seemed to have started sometime after starting your weight loss journey.

b. If you are uncertain about being in one, it's always best to do a reset and err on the side of caution. A plateau is not a "switch" phenomenon. It's a gradual thing over time. It's best to start your journey from the highest point we can get your metabolism too.

4. Fixing the Plateau with the Reset

a. You will need to count your calories during your reset. If you have no experience of how to do this, I recommend My Fitness Pal and YouTube.

b. Slowly increase your calories by 100-200 every couple of days until you hit somewhere close to your estimated TEE (total energy expenditure). You can do it in stages per week.

    c. Pay attention to how you feel overall with the increase in calories. Be sure to document somewhere. You will likely begin to feel better regarding:
   i. Brain Fog
   ii. Energy/tiredness
   iii. Pooping schedule, aka changes in bowel movements from being less constipated.
    d. Weekly weigh-ins are crucial here. You will likely stay at the same weight or even begin to drop weight as you increase your caloric intake. Although some people begin to gain weight, unfortunately.
   i. If you start to gain weight during the reset:
      1. Slow down the rate at which you are increasing your calories.
      2. Go as pure Keto as you can, getting as close to 0 net carbs as possible.
      3. Start stage one of fasting below.
    e. You can do stage 1 fasting explained in the next step, but do not progress past stage one. We have to focus on the reset first!
    f. Keto is critical to minimize weight gain as we increase calorie intake.
    g. Resets can take 2–5 weeks, but the average is 3.

5. **Fasting**
    a. There are three stages and your goal is to get to stage 3
    b. Stage 1 – Time-restricted eating or intermittent(IF) – 16/8 Choose a 6-9 hour eating window that ends at least three hours before bed and 2 hours after you wake. Do this for a week or until it becomes easy, and you are ready to progress.
    c. Stage 2 – 24 hour fasting. In addition to the above, add two 24-hour fasts per week. Every 3 days or so.

Even if you can't get to 24 hours on your first attempt, anything longer than the above is a win! Beat your time on the next one. This is the most difficult challenge for most people. Utilizing the support described in this book is crucial for many to break this point.

d. Stage 3 FLOA – 48 hours once per week. Same mentality as above. Even on the medications and/or peptides, you may not be able to get into the 48 your first time. Document how long you lasted and beat it next week ☺

e. Get enough calories on the non-long fasting days; aka eat near your TEE. I can't stress this enough! If you fast for 48 hours and then under-eat the following days, you will hit a plateau, and you will hit it fast! Gauge your intake compared to how you were eating 7 days per week before starting the program. You are to eat a minimum of that much for the five days but focusing on the better choices. This is mainly an issue for people that are on the GLP-1 medications like Semaglutide and/or Tirzepatide.

6. Fasting for women
   a. Avoid stages 2 and the FLOA stage of fasting during the 10 days before your period. Pay attention to how you feel during these 10 days regarding your fasting length for stage one. If you feel like crap when fasting from premenstrual symptoms, then you need to decrease the length of fasting. Some women cannot fast at all during this stage. Going keto during these days may also be challenging. More on this later!

7. Exercise
   a. Resistance training! This is your number one form of workout over any type of cardiovascular training. A

24

simple 3-day routine on non-fasting days is a great start. If you have little experience in this realm, then a personal trainer for 5–10 sessions with the goal of gaining comfort around your gym is great.

b. If you want to get extra workouts in, the best form is a special type of HIIT workout. See Appendix for this style.

8. Once you start your 24+ hour fasting

a. Add 1/8 tsp of Celtic or pink Himalayan salt 2x/day to these long fasting days. Anything past that 16-hour fasting period.

b. Take your normal supplements/medications as usual. Figure out how your body best handles them on an empty stomach, if any issue at all. You can take it with coffee and sugar-free non-dairy creamer. My favorite brand is Nut Pods. If it's still an issue, try soaking chia seeds in water overnight and take a spoonful with your supplements. Over time, it will get easier to take on an empty stomach.

   i. Consult your physician regarding any medication that requires food.

c. Coffee, tea, water, electrolytes, extra salt, vitamins, fish oil, stevia, monk fruit, erythritol, and a splash of Nut Pods creamer are allowed. NOTHING ELSE IS ALLOWED.

d. Take your salt and electrolytes every long fasting day.

e. Break your fast with smaller, easier-to-digest foods for a full day afterward before resuming normal intake. Bone broth soup is a great way to break it.

   i. See appendix for a list of suggested food options for breaking fast.

9. Keys to eating on non-fasting days

a. Ensure you are eating enough on the non-fasting days!!! If you don't count calories, then compare the volume of food to what normal was in the past. Or count for a few weeks just to get an idea.

b. You will likely have to separate yourself from your body in terms of hunger cues if you are on the GLP-1 medication. Since the Semaglutide/Tirzepatide is so powerful, you will not be hungry enough to eat what you have to eat to prevent a plateau on these days!

c. Calorie counting is optional. If it does not stress you out, It can be helpful, but not required for most people to be successful.

d. Follow the 90/10 for healthy food vs. cheat food ratio. Alcohol is a cheat.

10. Survive the fasting

a. Medications and/or appetite-suppressing supplement options to support

b. Mind set will be key here. Make a game for yourself to beat your time every time.

c. You will not die. Hunger is not a sign of damage to the body. In fact, you will grow stronger by overriding this feeling.

11. Hitting your goal! AKA, this is the FLOA lifestyle

a. Transition off the medications if you are using them, and keep the weekly FLOA fasting going.

b. Decrease the frequency to every other week for a few weeks.

c. As long as your weight is stable, continue to decrease to one of the following examples

d. 48 hours once every 2–4 weeks or 72 hours once every 3–6 weeks. The body loves variability. A long

26

fast at whatever frequency is maintaining a balance of weight for you.

e. Intermittent Fasting aka time restricted on other days as well.

f. Consistent weight training program.

g. Your 90/10 approach towards diet/junk can slip down to 85/15 or 80/20 if you desire. You need to learn how quickly your body slips back and find a balance that works for you!

Part One:
Why is it so damn difficult to lose weight and keep it off?

Why is it so hard for the majority of us to lose weight and keep it off?! Over the past 50 years, weight loss success has been a challenge for many individuals. In the United States, more than 20% of adults are now obese, and weight loss was not particularly successful even 50 years ago, with a 5% long-term success rate in conventional weight management (1). We have been taught to believe that one simply needs to exercise more and eat less, to lose weight, yet it has produced very little long-term results. Obese people have been made to feel inferior and inadequate. That it is solely their fault. But genetic studies paint a different picture. And within the people who have been successful long term; there appears to be this universal concept of wondering why it's always so much effort to maintain. I also personally experienced this.

Over the past 10 years, obesity rates have been increasing globally. In the United States, it is estimated that by 2030, 70% of the world's population of children and adolescents will be obese (2). In 2017, the Commission on Ending Childhood Obesity (ECHO) reported that worldwide obesity increased 10-fold among children and adolescents during the past 40 years.(3) This is scary stuff indeed. I believe the main problem is that the experts are not looking in the right place. To have an effective treatment approach, we have to understand what the hell is really going on to begin with. What are the mechanisms that are driving weight gain to begin with? But first, let's take a deeper dive and explore why it's been so difficult for us so far.

The Heavy Price: Obesity's Impact on our Health and Lives

Obesity has a significant impact on health and is associated with numerous serious diseases and health conditions. People with obesity are at an increased risk for:

1. All-causes of death (mortality) (4).
2. High blood pressure (hypertension) (5).
3. High LDL cholesterol, low HDL cholesterol, or high levels of triglycerides (dyslipidemia) (5).
4. Type 2 diabetes. (5).
5. Coronary heart disease (5).
6. Stroke (5).
7. Gallbladder disease.(5).
8. Some cancers, such as endometrial, breast, and colon cancer (5).
9. Osteoarthritis (5).
10. Gout (5).
11. Depression (5).
12. Obstructive sleep apnea (5)

These health issues can lead to long-term suffering, disability, and a reduced quality of life for individuals and their families. Additionally, obesity and its associated health problems have a significant economic impact on healthcare systems. It is important to note that the risk of health issues starts even when someone is only slightly overweight, and the likelihood of issues increases as someone becomes more overweight. This is because the deeper into the hole you get, the harder and harder it is to dig yourself out.

A body mass index (BMI) over 25 is considered overweight, and it increases the risk of various health issues. Some of the health concerns associated with being overweight include:

1. Increased risk of all-causes of death (mortality) (6)
2. Higher likelihood of developing high blood pressure (hypertension) (6).
3. Greater chance of having high LDL cholesterol, low HDL cholesterol, or high levels of triglycerides (dyslipidemia) (6).
4. Elevated risk of type 2 diabetes (6)
5. Higher risk of coronary heart disease (6).
6. Increased risk of stroke (6).
7. Greater likelihood of developing gallbladder disease (7).
8. Increased risk of certain cancers, such as endometrial, breast, and colon cancer (6).
9. Higher risk of developing osteoarthritis.
10. Greater chance of developing gout (8).
11. Increased risk of depression (8).
12. Higher likelihood of developing obstructive sleep apnea (8)

Being overweight can also have a negative impact on one's mental health. Research has shown that individuals with excess weight are at a higher risk of developing various mental health issues, including depression, anxiety, and eating disorders (9). Some possible reasons for this connection include:

1. Social stigma and discrimination: Overweight individuals often face social stigma and discrimination, which can lead to feelings of isolation, low self-esteem, and increased stress (10).
2. Hormonal imbalances: Obesity can contribute to hormonal imbalances, which may affect mood and increase the risk of anxiety and depression (9).
3. Physical health issues: Overweight individuals are at a higher risk of developing various health problems, which can contribute to feelings of stress, anxiety, and depression (11).

4. Lifestyle factors: Overeating, poor food choices, and a sedentary lifestyle, which are often associated with being overweight, can also contribute to mental health issues (12)

The social stigma that overweight and obese people receive is awful. You need to push all that crap aside and not let it affect you. This is important for mental health. It's good to not let yourself be impacted by how others may attempt to make you feel. There is a slippery slope through accepting yourself. The less you let yourself become impacted, the more potential you are to not see it as a big enough concern to take action and handle the issue. Hence, the slippery slope I mention. I'm not saying being depressed and frustrated so that it can fuel your changes is the ideal scenario. But I am saying that not acting on it is also not acceptable cither. When I was 16 I can admit it was being in the low point in my life that motivated my change. The most ideal scenario is keeping a strong mental space regarding your opinion about yourself and not let that be impacted by others. And at the same time, also understating the detrimental effects of being overweight so that you can take the necessary action for the right reasons. That would be a home run, for sure. If only we can all be this strong, right!?

Whatever it takes for you to get the job done and get your health in order before it gets worse is what I recommend for you. I share this information in this chapter with you to hopefully inspire you if you aren't in the obese category. Maybe you are only 15 pounds overweight, for example. Now you see the health ramifications of even a little extra weight. The biggest takeaway I want you to understand is this: every pound of fat that you pack on over your optimal weight/body fat percentage increases your inflammation and pushes you more into the insulin resistant pathway. In other words, it will become harder to get yourself out of it and back to a healthy state the more and more you push it off to the side. So quit kicking the can down the road, pick that sh** up already and take action. Speaking of action, let's get on to the solutions!

Betting on Yourself: How to Win with a Bad Hand

On Jan 1st, 2023, an episode on 60 minutes aired talking about obesity. An obesity expert by the name of Dr. Fatima Cody-Standford discussed how obesity is a "brain disease." She explains that very little could be done about the disease in terms of lifestyle choices. Next they showed a patient who is a gleaming example of someone who has the disease and cannot lose weight, despite her efforts. The rest of the show is talking about the new miracle weight loss medications; Wegovy. Many critics call this a glorified advertisement for Norvo Nordisk, the pharmaceutical company who designed and released Wegovy, the miracle drug in question. Yours truly is one of them. Dr. Apovian was the other doctor on the show, expressing her emphatic endorsement of Wegovy. Both Dr. Standord and Dr. Apovian advised on development of Wegovy and other obesity medications. They were both paid over $10,000 each in 2021 by Norvo Nordisk. I don't think this is an egregious amount to be paid for their work. What I found egregious though was 60 minutes not mentioning any of that in the show. For a TV show that supposedly prides itself in real investigative style reporting; it's obvious what agenda the show was accommodating.

I do indeed consider genetics heavily at play behind the obesity epidemic but consider this:

Genetics loads the gun, but lifestyle pulls the trigger.

You may have seen this quote touted by experts who put more weight on the environmental side of the nature vs. nurture debate. I don't think it's so black and white, though. Genetics regarding any disease carry a particular percentage of contribution to the development and progression of said condition. While we can study diseases and learn more about how genetically based they are in nature, it's important to understand two concepts: much less can be done about the genetic part, and individual variability will also exist.

Regarding obesity, we can look at a few studies to better understand the heavy amount of genetic contribution. Adoptive families are good to look at. Here, you have children raised by parents with no genetic relation but 100% environmental exposure. Dr. Albert J. Stunkard performed classic studies on obesity by looking at 540 Danish adult adoptees. No relationship whatsoever was found between parents and adoptees in terms of weight. When they compared them to their biological parents, the opposite was discovered. A strong correlation was found with the biological parents. The results say a lot about the genetic basis for obesity. Another classic type of study is to look at twins, both identical and fraternal. Dr. Stunkard did just that; he also accounted for them being reared together or apart and compared weights to isolate how specifically that environment played a role. He concluded that about 70% of obesity and weight issues are controlled by genetics. This was a giant discovery that unfortunately failed to influence much of how we have been approaching obesity.

Science has even identified multiple genes contributing to an individual's susceptibility to obesity. The fat mass and obesity-associated (FTO) gene is one of the well-known genes associated with obesity. Other genes, such as RIPK1 and VDR, have also been implicated in some studies. The interaction between genetic factors and environmental influences, such as physical activity, can also play a role in the development of obesity.(13)

Is this enough evidence to justify what 60 minutes portrayed? In my opinion….. No. The show really leaves you feeling like it's 100%

genetics, and therefore, you can't blame yourself if you have this disease. There are some real "incurable" genetically based diseases, for sure. The 60-minute show leaves you feeling like nothing at all can be done and not to blame yourself whatsoever. With that mentality, one begins to take less and less responsibility for one's condition of obesity. Sadly, this mindset ultimately leads to more and more weight gain, of course. In my opinion, it's important to understand that you may have been dealt a crappy hand, but to understand that you can do something about it. According to 60 minutes, though; hey...... It's okay, folks, we have your only solution to this genetic "disease," and that's lifelong adherence to the new drug.

We have our cholesterol, blood pressure, and diabetes medications that we would never consider stopping due to the nature of these irreversible diseases. Now, we have our obesity medication. ~Dr. Jones DC

How many "chronic diseases" will we have by 2030 that will necessitate lifelong adherence to medication? The marketing tactics of big pharmaceuticals are powerful. Every day, I converse with people who 100% bought into this mindset of obesity being an incurable disease that requires pharmacological treatment for life. I understand part of why they feel that way. Millions have tried their best to battle this issue. But we have been taught the wrong information. It's always been a losing battle for us. With our patients, we provide the medications to help jumpstart the program and break the initial barriers that obese individuals struggle with. Our program emphasizes powerful strategies that allow patients to ultimately ween off the medications and sustain their weight. We will dive into all of that later on.

I educate the public across various social media platforms advocating this very idea of weaning off medications being a potential reality, for some. In response, I receive many comments that generally sound like this: "You wouldn't tell someone to stop their blood pressure medication, would you? So why would you advocate getting off these medications?" I generally respond with something like, "Would you continue to take blood pressure medication if you no longer needed to take it to maintain a healthy blood pressure?" While ½ of them get frustrated and defensive, the other 1⁄2 may end up wanting to learn more. Some people really were just dealt a crappy hand because of their genetics; there is no denying this fact. But there is hope. Millions of people have reversed their obesity and transformed their health. We have had the pleasure of helping thousands ourselves. Let's take a brief history lesson and see if we can learn something from it.

Let History Teach us Something

Obesity Is not something you saw in the pre-industrial area. The more and more industrialized we become, the greater the incidence of obesity we begin to see. Evolutionarily speaking, it would be rather difficult to become obese with the great deal of effort it took to secure the next meal. Times undeniably have changed now, and so has the occurrence of obesity. By the late 1800s, it was accepted that excessive consumption of refined carbs was the main culprit behind obesity. For the next 100 years, lowering the consumption of these types of food was the standard of treatment for obesity. Just ask your grandparents what they did back in the day to treat obesity. It's rather amusing to think that the Atkins and Keto craze was something that already existed and was well understood over 100 years ago.

Something changed in the 1950s, though. Heart disease rates were increasing at an alarming rate. The public was concerned and experts were looking for answers. Little did they realize there was a very rational explanation for this increase. At that time, increases in vaccines, modern medicine such as antibiotics and increased public health measures dramatically decreased deaths due to infections. Naturally, this would then lead to more opportunities to die from heart disease. It's just a simple result of living longer. Life expectancies were about 15 years longer after these changes, which brought the life expectancy to about mid-60s. That is about the time when heart disease tends to set in. Unfortunately, they did not make the connection then because they blamed something that ultimately led to the beginning of a worldwide epidemic.

What they blamed was fat. Fat is the villain causing all the heart attacks, they said. All they had to lean on was some questionable research connecting dietary fat intake with increased cholesterol levels and their perceived roles in heart disease. While many pointed to fat and cholesterol, some denied this. Using logic here, how could fat suddenly start causing heart attacks if it didn't before? We observed refined carb intake makes us gain weight, and its restriction produces reliable weight loss. We knew that for the last 100 years! How were they now, all of a sudden, no longer a problem? When you reduce fat intake, you have to replace the calories, and the only categories left are carbs and protein. Eating all protein wasn't a reality, leaving us with only carbs. So it must be calories, they said, not the carbs! That's the only way to make sense of what they proposed and what we knew from history. Calories, fat, and cholesterol are the concerns they proclaimed. For the next 20 years, great debate existed about the true culprit of obesity. That ended with the government deciding for us.

One historic day in 1977, the US Committee on Nutrition chairman declared that diets high in fat and total calories were the real concerns that must be handled. This set forth the dietary guidelines for the USA. Please understand that there was no monumental

36

discovery in the science of obesity. There was nothing conclusive or anything close that they could lean on to justify this radical policy change, just the government making the final health call for us. This is the first time in history that Big Brother decided on our health. And boy, did they get this horribly wrong. Massive efforts rolled out across the USA to change our approach towards nutrition. They changed everything they could to get us to adopt this new approach. This is where the food pyramid came from, that we all grew up learning about as a kid. The one that told us we needed most of our calories to come from carbs.

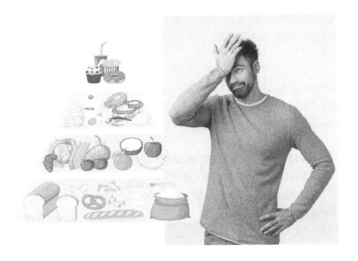

Yes, that one. All the health agencies jumped on board, and anyone who advocated against these ideas was ostracized. When browsing old guidelines, the ones from the American Heart Association make me chuckle the most. In the mid-1990s, they advocated a diet that allowed white bread and carbonated beverages. In case you guys didn't know, the president of the American Health Association(AHA), John Warner, had a heart attack in the fall of 2017. He has a family history of heart disease, though, so I'm sure the AHA guidelines helped the 52-year-old not get a heart attack much earlier in his life, right?

So, the people did as they were told. Fat intake was reduced from 45% to 35%, and egg consumption decreased by 18%. As explained earlier, a decrease in fat intake means an inevitable increase in carb consumption. And we were now striving to consume about 60% of our caloric information in grains and pasta. Do you remember your daily school lunches? Sandwiches with white bread, chips or crackers, high sugar fruit cups of some sort, chocolate milk or juice, and don't forget the sweet treat for dessert. Adults more conscious of their health tried to be healthy and bought fat-free foods to lower their fat intake. We all drank the proverbial Kool-Aid.

Heart disease got better, yea? With this massive shift to reduce fat, calories, and cholesterol paired with increased exercise; it had to get somewhat better, right? No, it certainly did not get better.

But something else sure happened due to the changes Big Brother ordered us to make. Rates of obesity and, eventually, skyrocketing rates of diabetes followed. See the chart below to look at the year obesity exploded.

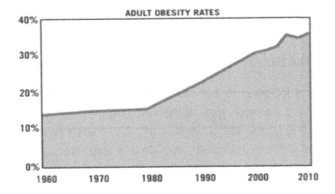

Chart Data from National Health and Nutrition Examination Survey (NHANES) (14)

You can see a slight and steady increase in obesity each decade. Something that makes sense to me with the advancements in technology that require less physical work, and increased access to fast foods and processed foods. But look at that sharp change in the angle of the graph. It's scary how pinpointed that increase is. Right around the same year, Big Brother stepped in and called for us to change our dietary guidelines. There are certainly many things we can point the finger at. The explosion of fast food restaurants, increased technology developments that foster less activity, increases in the % of processed foods versus whole foods, and many more could be considered. It is firmly in my opinion that there is a common denominator here. That is the shift to a carb-rich diet with emphasis on snacking throughout the day. There is no coincidence in the timing of the stark increase in obesity rates and the massive changes in our diet. What do carbs and snacking do that make us so obese? We will explain this in the upcoming chapters. But first, let's look at what else we have been taught to believe that has contributed to why it's been so damn difficult to get in shape.

Breaking the Rules: When What We Learned Was Wrong

Science is supposed to be constantly evolving. More and more questions are asked that either strengthen or weaken our understanding of the way things work. As a result of the massive shift in our dietary approach, we clearly impacted the onset of obesity; there is no denying this. Increased carb intake and emphasis on snacking are affecting us in ways that are making us more obese. We will discuss the mechanics of all that in the upcoming chapters. But first let's look at some strong opinions we have held onto and still hold on to that are not helping us either.

Eating six meals a day will "rev up" your metabolism

The concept of eating six small meals throughout the day has been debated for centuries, with some cultures believing in the benefits of a single meal per day, while others promote a "nibbling diet" of 17 snacks per day. The premise behind eating smaller and more frequent meals is the control of blood sugar, also called blood glucose. This refers to the glucose, a type of sugar that is extracted from the food we eat. When digestion is complete, glucose is carried by the bloodstream and throughout the body to provide energy for various cellular processes. Eating smaller meals more frequently can help regulate blood sugar levels, preventing spikes and crashes that can lead to feelings of hunger and overeating. The problem here is that every time you eat, you have to release insulin to bring your blood sugar down. You will learn later about how detrimental to weight loss the presence of insulin in the bloodstream is.

The thermic effect of food (TEF) is the energy we expend to process, use, and store the nutrients in our meals. However, the temporary boost in our metabolic rates is directly proportional to how much and what types of foods we eat. So, while eating six small meals over the course of a day would slightly increase your metabolism six times, eating three larger meals per day can result in a similar overall effect through three proportionally larger boosts.(15)

Breakfast like a king, lunch like a prince, dinner like a peasant.

The concept of "eating breakfast like a king, lunch like a prince, and dinner like a peasant" suggests that we should consume our largest meal in the morning, a moderate-sized meal for lunch, and a smaller meal for dinner. This idea has been passed down through generations and is often associated with promoting weight loss and overall health. In blue zones regions, where people tend to live longer and healthier lives, a similar routine is followed, with a focus on consuming the majority of the day's calories before noon.(16) The reasoning behind this concept is rooted in the idea that our metabolism is most active earlier in the day and slows down as the day progresses. By front-loading our calories and consuming a substantial breakfast, we are providing our bodies with the energy it needs for the day ahead. Additionally, eating a lighter dinner can help prevent overeating and promote better digestion during sleep

So we clearly understand the negative health consequences of eating more of your calories closer to bed and how that hinders weight loss efforts. But aside from this fact, the rest of it provides no extra benefit. You do not need to fuel yourself every single morning to have energy for the day. Our bodies are wonderful at running off stored energy in many forms. The largest reservoir of stored energy is body fat. This also plays into the whole 6 meals per day nonsense; the body has evolved survival mechanisms beyond needing to eat so often. Survival wouldn't look so good otherwise, now would it? You have a daily requirement of calories to consume if the goal is to maintain weight, but for the rest of us here who need to lose weight. Tapping into the very mechanisms of survival is not only more effective but way healthier for you as well!

Breakfast is the most important meal of the day

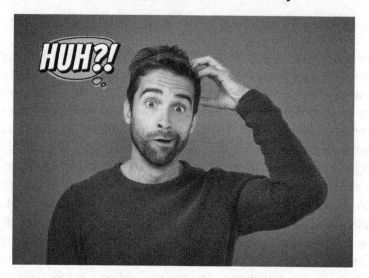

This concept truthfully shows the power of marketing and its ability to impinge on a society and persist through time; despite science telling us that it makes no sense at all. Here is the thing, when you wake up each morning, your body actually feeds you already!

Diabetics call this the "Dawn Phenomenon." This is where they find their sugars are actually higher in the morning. The body operates on a clock called the circadian rhythm, and this clock times the release of specific hormones that cause the liver to dump out sugar into the bloodstream. From an evolutionary perspective, it makes a lot of sense to provide energy for you to start the day and not need to take time to eat

Just think about it for a minute; how often do you really wake up hungry? You don't because there is already a rise in blood sugar from the food you ate yesterday. Yet, the majority of us have carried this idea that you need to "fuel the start of your day." But hey, you can keep listening to the big breakfast companies like Kellogg's. ☺ It's important to understand that some people feel worse throughout the day when they skip breakfast. We're not talking about true Hypoglycemics or Diabetics who have medical issues which can let them slip into dangerously low levels of blood sugar that could be fatal. But outside these extremes, there are many who "feel" better when they eat a hearty breakfast. How do we make sense of this observation?

I like to explain it like this. Imagine you have a rusty chainsaw that's been sitting in your garage for decades. When you go to use it, it will likely not work or if it does, will not run efficiently. We have two sides of our metabolism, the fat burning side and the carb burning side. The fat burning system is there to sustain us and keep us alive during times of famine. Hence, the large amount of body fat we can store on our body. Your body produces ketone bodies as an alternative source of fuel in the absence of carbs. Ketone bodies actually produce a "heightened sense." This is why you have heard people speak of feeling more energetic and aware when fasting or on a keto diet. It makes a lot of evolutionary sense as well. If we felt like crap when we had no food, our chances of an effective hunt would not be as good. Most of us have rarely needed to use the fat burning side. So when you finally decide to use that system in your body; say, for example, start a fasting and/or ketogenic diet, your body goes wonky. Your brain needs a steady stream of energy. So when it detects lower amounts, such as the onset of this change in your diet, it starts to freak out. Just like that rusty chainsaw that doesn't work too well or at all, your body is very ineffective at supplying energy to itself at this point, and therefore you feel like crap. Once you lube up and reconfigure the chainsaw, it will work great again. The lube in this analogy would be the time it takes for that system to become efficient again.

It's all about calories in vs. out

Finally, the old calories in vs. calories out concept. I will save the science on why this doesn't work for upcoming chapters. But every robust large-scale study that utilized an approach consisting of restricting calories and increasing exercise all failed to demonstrate long-term success. The majority regained it back. A common-sense observation by many of you reading this now. How many times have you cut your calories, lost some weight, and struggled to keep it off? Calories matter, yes, but without understanding of rest and how to approach it, we clearly cannot solve the problem. Once you understand the rest, you realize they matter much less than you can possibly imagine!

Obesity: The Current State of Affairs

According to the Centers for Disease Control and Prevention (CDC) the age-adjusted prevalence of obesity among U.S. adults was 42.4% in 2017–2018. The prevalence was 40.0% among younger adults aged 20–39, 44.8% among middle-aged adults aged 40–59, and 42.8% among older adults aged 60 and over. The age-adjusted prevalence of severe obesity was 9.2% among adults aged 20 and over in the United States in 2017–2018. The overall prevalence of obesity was similar among men and women, but the prevalence of severe obesity was higher among women. Adults aged 40–59 had the highest prevalence of severe obesity (17).

44

Globally, the prevalence of obesity nearly tripled between 1975 and 2016. According to the World Health Organization (WHO) in 2016, more than 1.9 billion adults, 18 years and older, were overweight. Of these, over 650 million were considered to be affected by obesity (BMI ≥30 kg/m²), which equates to 39% of men and 40% of women of adults aged 18 or over living with overweight and 13% living with obesity.(6) The World Obesity Federation estimates that by 2020 around 770 million adults globally will be affected by obesity, and that figure is anticipated to exceed one billion by 2030 unless we act soon. (18)

Obesity is a growing problem in children and adolescents as well. From 1975 to 2016, the prevalence of overweight or obese children and adolescents aged 5–19 years increased more than four-fold, from 4% to 18% globally. The vast majority of overweight or obese children live in developing countries, where the rate of increase has been more than 30% higher than that of developed countries.(19). Obesity in childhood is associated with a wide range of serious health complications and an increased risk of premature onset of related illnesses

In the United States, the obesity prevalence was 41.9% in 2017 – March 2020 From 1999 to 2000 through 2017 –March 2020, US obesity prevalence increased from 30.5% to 41.9%. During the same time, the prevalence of severe obesity increased from 4.7% to 9.2%.(18) Obesity-related conditions include heart disease, stroke, type 2 diabetes, and certain types of cancer. These are among the leading causes of preventable, premature death. The estimated annual medical cost of obesity in the United States was nearly $173 billion in 2019 dollars, Medical costs for adults who were obese were $1,861 higher than medical costs for people with a healthy weight.

Societal views on obesity

In today's society, overweight individuals face significant challenges and negative perceptions due to societal views on obesity. These views have a profound impact on their lives, impacting their personal well-being, social interactions, and overall health. Here are some of the ways this is happening:

1. Negative beliefs and stereotypes: Modern society has adopted negative beliefs about obese individuals, often perceiving them as lazy, irresponsible, and lacking self-discipline. These stereotypes overlook the complex nature of obesity, which is influenced by genetic, socioeconomic, and environmental factors. The media plays a role in perpetuating these negative attitudes by depicting thin actors as popular and kind, while overweight actors are often portrayed as rude, aggressive, and unpopular.

2. Weight stigma: Weight stigma is prevalent in various domains of society, including the media, schools, workplaces, and even healthcare settings. Overweight individuals may face discrimination, prejudice, and bias due to their weight. This stigma can lead to negative consequences such as disordered eating, decreased physical activity, and psychological distress.

3. Media portrayal: The media plays a significant role in shaping societal views on obesity. Television shows and movies typically depict overweight characters as unattractive, unintelligent, unhappy, and cruel. This portrayal reinforces negative stereotypes and contributes to weight stigma. Furthermore, news images that focus on body parts or emphasize weight can dehumanize individuals with obesity.

4. Impact on children: Even children's programs and movies communicate negative messages about being overweight. Overweight cartoon characters are typically depicted as unattractive, unintelligent, and unhappy. This can lead to the internalization of weight bias among children and perpetuate weight stigma into adulthood.

5. Healthcare bias: Unfortunately, weight stigma also exists in healthcare settings. Healthcare professionals, including physicians, nurses, dietitians, psychologists, and medical students, have been found to hold negative attitudes towards individuals with excess weight. This bias can result in inappropriate treatment and hinder the healthcare of obese individuals.

The consequences of societal views on obesity are significant. They can have a detrimental impact on the lives of overweight individuals. I grew up experiencing a lot of bullying and teasing because of my weight, so I know how bad it can be and how badly it made me feel. Now that I understand the genetic component of obesity, I much more appreciate what I had to personally go through and, more importantly, why it is such a tall order for more to accomplish. We need a more profound understanding of this as a society to foster the improvements that we so desperately need as obesity continues to get worse and worse.

What Does it Mean to be Sustainable?

Diets are often thought of as a quick-fix for weight loss, but the reality is that most diets fail in the long term. The literature has shown this many times. I'm sure you have personally experienced many rounds of weight loss followed by weight gain over time. There are several reasons why this is the case, and understanding these reasons is crucial for anyone looking to lose weight and actually keep it off. In this chapter, I will focus on the lack of sustainability regarding current weight loss solutions available.

What does it mean to be sustainable? The effort that you took to lose the weight is one thing. But the effort required to maintain the weight loss has to be something you can honestly maintain. It has to be practical. Let's say we can quantify effort on a scale of 1-100. You have 100 units of effort to spend on various parts of your life. You always have 100 no matter what. Life will always ebb and flow. It's one thing to get super serious and use up 50% of your effort towards this goal for say 3 months. But for how long can you keep this up? Even the most disciplined will eventually experience life getting in the way and eventually fall off the bandwagon.

To be successful in the long term, it is crucial to focus on making sustainable changes to your eating habits from the start, rather than putting in maximal effort. I'm not here to shame maximal effort. I love high levels of enthusiasm towards lifestyle changes; and really toward goal accomplishment in general. But we have to be honest with ourselves when talking about weight loss. And what percentage of effort can we and are we willing to maintain for the rest of our lives?

The biggest problems I have with weight loss programs are not their success towards initial weight loss. But what we require is a program that actually empowers us to carry over the habits necessary to **MAINTAIN THE WEIGHT LOSS!** You can call these habits or I like to think of them more as an operating basis. The only thing more frustrating than not being able to lose weight, is losing weight and regaining it back. And trust me when I say I speak from experience. As you recall from earlier, I yo-yoed in personal weight for years. It's pretty depressing and frustrating at the same time.

So, how does one maintain the weight loss they have recently achieved? This is the part that weight loss programs seem to talk about much less than they should. That's because it would initially appear that the amount of effort it takes to maintain your weight loss is less than actually losing the weight itself. From a physical calorie burning and calorie consumption standpoint, this is true. But what's interesting about this is when you begin to think about the mindset during weight loss. When you are actively losing weight; you are likely experiencing a "high". Look; we are not talking about losing a couple of pounds here. I doubt many of you would be reading this book otherwise. When your goal is, for example, 10% or more of your body weight, and you are actively achieving consistent weight loss towards this goal, you begin to develop this "high." You are seeing the fruits of your labor and the feeling is f****** fantastic to say the least. The amount of effort it takes and level of dedication it takes to continue to lose the weight starts to decrease. It starts to feel more natural and "effortless" because you are so pumped about the results.

It's because of this, that while it appears to be more "effort" to lose weight than simply maintaining it..... Many experience the opposite. Including yours truly.

So you lose your 20lbs, and you feel very wonderful and rewarded and happy and yada yada yada. You should feel this way..... You earned it. But the high phases out, and before you know it, you are back to the normal game of life. You aren't fixated on the results anymore. Eventually, you stop staring at yourself in the mirror. Yes, they noticed this habit of yours.

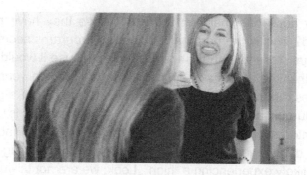

Suddenly, that innate urge to stick to your "clean eating" or saying "no, thank you" to the polite and also skinny coworker who brought donuts for everyone becomes much harder than it was before. Suddenly, you find it harder and harder to say no to your friends and/or family who want to get together because you need to go to the gym instead. Waking up to go to the gym before work at the crack of dawn now feels twice as hard. WHAT THE HELL? This is precisely why I think the "maintaining weight loss" part is much harder than the "losing it" part.

Essentially, you have to continue with the changes to your normal operating basis that you did during the weight loss, but without the "high" that made it so much easier. And yes, you should need less physical effort to maintain it. But even with this fact, it's challenging for many to maintain. Thinking of all the people you know who lost more than 10% of their body weight, how many of them kept it off for good?

You have to incorporate some amount of change to the way you operate your life PERMANENTLY. Meaning; keep doing some of those things you did to lose the weight even after the fact. And the only changes you have recently learned are the ones that you did to lose the weight to begin with. If the changes that you did to lose the weight are overbearing, time-consuming, stressful, tedious etc., then you are likely setting yourself up for failure. Unfortunately, life ebbs and flows and commitments that at earlier times were possible can unexpectedly become difficult. The only way I feel confident communicating to patients about a way to confidently minimize this risk of weight regain is if the effort it took to lose the weight initially was, itself, less effort to begin with. If, for example, it only took 25-40% of our available effort rather than the customary 50%. This gives us more wiggle room to be able to handle those unexpected stresses in the future while still maintaining the effort it requires to stay in shape.

Out of all the popular methods of weight loss out there, the common theme I see is the old tried and true calorie reduction method. The exception to this, of course, is the keto/Atkins, and we will discuss that one later.

Why Reducing Calories Never Works

Reducing calories has been at the center of the government's war on obesity for decades. Billions of dollars have been spent on numerous programs that emphasized reduction of calories and increases in exercise. The overwhelming consensus is that this method will yield results initially, but ultimately, there is always the point where people begin to regain their weight. Why why why? Are people simply weak-minded and unable to refrain from overeating themselves back to prior weights? I'm sure you can say that's the case for some people. You would think having your doctors tell you to eat less and exercise more for all those years would have helped, right? Why do we see so many doctors themselves overweight? They understand the science of calories in vs. calories out and presumably have the finances to afford better food options; a luxury many cannot. Yet, they seem to struggle almost as much as anyhow else? Let's take a closer look at the calorie.

The calorie is the measurement of energy used when we discuss human physiology. There are nine calories in a gram of fat and four calories in a gram of either protein or carbs. Our bodies require a certain number of calories to function. All the various physiological processes in the body require calories to run, so as a whole the body requires a total sum of calories. We refer to this measurement as the Resting Metabolic Rate or RMR. Then we need to account for the amount of activity one does every day, as this can obviously range from very sedentary to high amounts of activity for say a physical laboring job. When we account for this activity, we call this figure the total energy expenditure or TEE. The basic premise is this: eat less than this number of calories, and you will lose weight, and consume more than this, and you will gain weight. While this fact appears to be true at face value, there is clearly more going on. Our global campaigns to eat less would have yielded some better results otherwise. There have been some assumptions regarding calories and weight loss that we seem to still latch onto. Let's dissect these

Calories in vs. out have no effect on each other

Numerous journals have demonstrated a change in the number of calories burned by the body in reaction to a change in the consumption. And it goes both ways, up and down. This demonstrates that your BMR is not static, but can change due to various reasons.(1) What causes these changes?

We control caloric intake

Tell that to the dieters who experience ravenous hunger when dieting. You know that feeling, as you have likely reduced your calories in the past. That hunger you experienced was noticeably higher when on your diet, wasn't it? Do you control your hunger, or does your hunger control you? We'd like to think the former, but the truth about hunger is that its activity is governed and controlled by both the nervous and endocrine systems. What regulates the overall feeling of hunger that ultimately dictates caloric intake?

Fat stores are unregulated

Do we simply lose weight or gain weight at the rate of the caloric deficit or surplus we produce through diet and exercise? There are many hormones like leptin and insulin that tightly regulate weight gain and loss. They clearly act independent of calories. Just look at a type 1 diabetic, for example. They literally cannot gain weight despite how much they eat until they are diagnosed and begin treatment with insulin.

All calories are the same

We all inherently know that eating 2000 calories of Snickers bars vs. eating 2000 calories of broccoli would yield different results, yet we still latch on to this calorie ideal being the very senior rule above all else. So what governs how the body reacts to the various forms of calories?

Calorie reduction is not the primary factor in weight loss. The literature has shown this many times through. The law of thermodynamics is commonly quoted when thinking of weight management in terms of calories in vs. out. "Energy cannot be created or destroyed in an isolated system" The reality is that the human body is a very complex system and therefore not isolated. We have numerous parts of the body that each require various amounts of energy. Hormones are responsible for regulating the allocation of calories towards the various systems. Imagine if it was actually static for a minute. Imagine if our ancestors, who experienced longer periods without food and had a BMR that didn't change? Survival looks very bleak, doesn't it? When you look at weight loss or weight gain in the extreme ends, the calories never add up. Research has shown decreases in BMR rates in reaction to calorie restriction over time. And if you look at the number of calories an obese person consumes and has consumed during their years of slow and steady weight gain, they should have gained weight much faster than they did.

How does the body accomplish such feats? It literally changes its metabolic rate and your level of hunger. You lose energy, get more foggy minded, poop less often and, over time, can even begin to lose hair. Meanwhile, you are trying to deal with levels of hunger that are now higher than ever before. Dieters can tell you how hungry they are and how little weight they seem to be losing despite the caloric deficit they think they are in. Even if they fought the hunger and maintained the lower intake of calories, they are actually burning fewer calories at rest now. Genius design for survival, horrible design for desired weight loss.

What about exercise? Exercise has amazing benefits for our health outside of weight management and should be done regularly because of this. But in terms of weight management, it unfortunately isn't much better than calorie restriction. We must understand the concept of a calorie deficit vs. a caloric surplus. The caloric deficit describes having burned more calories over a period of time than consumed. You can accomplish the deficit by eating less and/or exercising more. It is probably better for you, in theory, to rely more on the exercise side of that equation than the caloric restriction side because you can only restrict your calories so much. My point is that the body responds to the caloric deficit over time in the same fashion, regardless of how you got there.

The other thing about exercise to understand is that it requires time; a commodity that many have very little to allocate. Necessities and priorities always shift, as life will always throw curveballs. My patients have always been so shocked when they start with me and I have them exercise less than what they are used to. But in doing so, they many times maintain weight with no change in caloric intake, which would only be possible if the metabolism increased to offset the reduction of exercise. This really plays into the sustainability part of what I emphasize so much with the FLOA protocol. If you only have to exercise 3x a week rather than 6x a week, which one looks more sustainable to you? What do you feel more confident about committing too?

So our bodies are working against weight loss when we eat less and/or exercise more. What about attempts to gain weight? We see the same effect taking place. Research on both mice and humans demonstrates that the body will resist long-term weight gain in reaction to a consistent increase in calories. Seeing this work on both sides really drives this point. There exists an underlying mechanism in the body that desires to maintain homeostasis, aka some sort of balance. Again, imagine if the bodies didn't do this. Just pretend there were no systems at play to help regulate weight. That it's all a matter of numbers. This would not have obviously worked back when we didn't have the technology to even count/track calories. And now that we do today; I can honestly say

it's about 1% of people I have worked with that actually enjoyed counting calories. I mean truthfully enjoy it. In other words, they would still do it if they didn't have to!

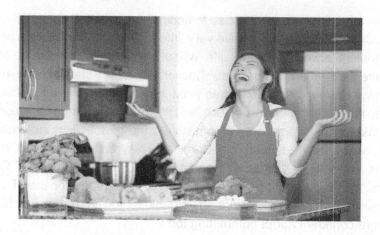

Most people are clueless about the number of calories they consume, and that's ok! I promise if you follow my program, you won't need to track calories, and you will have more time to enjoy life! We call this weight range that your body desires to maintain, a set point. Much like the thermostat of a house maintaining a certain temperature. Your body has a weight that it is literally striving to maintain. Areas in your brain, specifically in the hypothalamus, control this set point. This part of the brain also controls other basic functions such as sexual behavior, circadian rhythms and how you sleep, body temperature and various basic feelings. We can physically manipulate these tissues to pretty rapidly create obesity or massive weight loss. These manipulations would dramatically change metabolism and hunger, leading to rapid weight changes. There was an experiment in which scientists connected the blood supply between two mice, but they still maintained their separate brains and organ function. They then lesioned one of the rats in this same area of the brain in a way that they expected to produce obesity; and so it did. But what happened to the other rat was rather interesting. It actually lost a lot of weight.(1) Remember, it shares blood supply with the first rat.

Something in the blood was trying to fight the obesity created by the brain of the mouse made obese. This proves that there are things in the blood supply that play a major role in the onset of obesity.

The weight set point theory

The weight set point theory suggests that the human body has a specific weight range that it aims to maintain, and the body will adapt to keep that weight. This is accomplished through various compensatory physiological mechanisms to maintain this set point and resist deviation from it. When a person loses weight, these mechanisms drive the weight back to the set point, resulting in regaining the lost weight. Conversely, when someone gains weight, mechanisms drive the weight back down to the set point.(1) This concept certainly explains everything we have discussed thus far.

Multiple studies have demonstrated this fact. The idea that obese people have slow metabolisms has been proven wrong. In fact, many studies show they actually burn more calories.(6) Their bodies are attempting to resist weight gain. Think of the thermostat in your house. It's the master regulator of the temperature. If you were hot and brought in a small AC unit next to you, you would indeed cool off. But eventually the thermostat would sense the change and produce more heat until ultimately, you're back at the same temperature with the small AC unit running. In real-time, changes to your weight; you restrict your calories and/or increase your exercise to accomplish some amount of weight loss. Eventually, your weight loss plateaus. But now you are in a different environment than before the weight loss started. You are now eating less and/or exercising more with no weight change. Just like the thermostat bringing back the temperature to baseline with the portable AC unit being on now, your body acts in the same manner in regard to maintaining a certain weight.

So how do we change the thermostat naturally? Since surgical procedures to favorably manipulate the hypothalamus are out of the question, we must focus on what's left: hormones. How do we address the hormonal issues at play? To understand the solution, it helps to first understand the science of obesity.

Part Two:
Understanding the Science of Obesity

So you now have a much better comprehension of the practical reasons why it's been so challenging for you to drop weight and keep it off. Let's chalk it up to some bad luck for all of us. Not only are your genetics working against you, but you have also been taught to believe things that are just plain bad. Eating a higher percentage of carbs and snacking more often has been harmful to most of mankind; minus the big processed food corporations. Obesity is a condition in which the hormones are not properly regulating fat mass. They are in a state of dysregulation. What is very evident thus far is that there is a giant piece missing of our understanding of how all that works. That is why, as of today, we continue to look at the wrong solutions. Now, we need to get into the weeds of it all and look at the science behind what has been happening in our bodies this entire time. Only then will our radically genius solution, The FLOA protocol, begin to make a lot of sense.

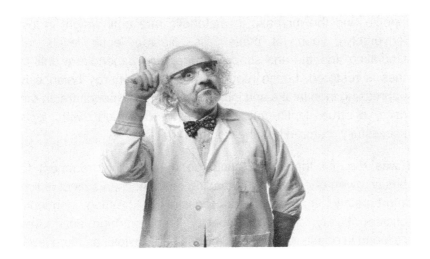

Hormonal Harmony: Insulin's Dominant Influence on Weight Management

A hormone is a chemical substance secreted by an endocrine gland or group of endocrine cells that acts to control or regulate specific physiological processes in the body. The endocrine system is simply our system of glands that produce the various hormones that affect most aspects of your body's functions. Hormones are produced in one part of the body and travel through the bloodstream to impact other parts of the body. They exert their effects on target cells or organs via specific receptors on the target cells.

What to understand about Leptin

The discovery of the hormone leptin and its role affecting the hypothalamus to regulate obesity was very promising. Leptin levels are directly proportional to the percentage of fat mass in the body. When fat mass increases, leptin levels increase. This is sensed by the hypothalamus, which then coordinates the suppression of appetite and the increase in metabolic rate until weight is lost. Conversely, when fat mass falls, plasma leptin levels fall, stimulating appetite and suppressing energy expenditure until fat mass is restored. Leptin regulates long-term energy balance by suppressing food intake and increasing energy expenditure. In rare cases of true leptin-deficient obesity, treatment with leptin successfully restored healthy weight. (20)

It was thought that leptin could be a promising treatment for obesity, given our new understanding of its mechanisms of action. Unfortunately, it proved unsuccessful at treating non-leptin deficient obesity, aka normal obesity. Turns out high leptin levels are found in obese individuals, which is paradoxical, as more leptin should cause the opposite. The only explanation for this is some

60

sort of resistance to leptin in obese individuals. We now understand leptin resistance to indeed exist. (21)

What about insulin?

Insulin plays a crucial role in regulating energy balance by controlling various metabolic processes in the body. It affects food intake, energy burning, and glucose metabolism in both tissues of the arms and legs, as well as the central nervous system. In the brain, insulin signaling has been implicated in the control of satiety and energy balance. Insulin acts on specific neurons in the hypothalamus, which is a key region involved in the regulation of energy balance. AKA Direct hormonal control over your hunger and metabolic rate. When insulin levels are high, it promotes glucose uptake into cells and inhibits the breakdown of fats, leading to a positive energy balance. On the other hand, when insulin levels are low, the body shifts towards utilizing stored energy in the form of glycogen (stored carbs) and fat, resulting in a negative energy balance. Insulin also interacts with other hormones, such as leptin, which plays a major role in regulating appetite and energy expenditure. Moreover, insulin has indirect effects on energy balance. For example, it suppresses fat mobilization, preventing the conversion of stored fats into free fatty acids, thereby making it harder for you to burn fat. Another indirect mechanism involves the inhibition of glucagon release from the pancreas, which results in reduced glucose output from the liver

Insulin levels clearly play multiple roles, ultimately affecting your propensity to gain weight or lose it. But does it stand up to the test? Does insulin cause you to gain weight? We are going to delve into the various mechanisms that are demonstrated by science.

Let's look at diabetics

Why do we see very different body types between type 1 and type 2 diabetics? What is the difference? The main difference between type 1 and type 2 diabetes lies in the causes and the way the body responds to insulin. Type 1 diabetes is an autoimmune disease in which the body's immune system attacks and destroys the insulin-producing cells in the pancreas. As a result, the body completely stops making insulin, and people with type 1 diabetes must take daily insulin injections or use an insulin pump to survive.

On the other hand, type 2 diabetes is caused by a resistance to insulin. It's the complete opposite scenario regarding insulin levels found in the blood. High levels of insulin are found in their bodies, but insulin's ability to lower blood sugar has decreased. In this case, the pancreas still produces insulin, but the body's cells become resistant to it, leading to elevated blood sugar levels. The pancreas tries to compensate by producing more insulin, but over time, it becomes less effective. More and more insulin is made to compensate, but it's the high levels of insulin itself creating more and more resistance. It's like a giant boulder rolling down a hill, building more and more momentum as it continues down, becoming harder and harder to stop.

Before the advancement of medicine and the availability of therapeutic insulin; the prognosis for type one diabetics was terrible. They would literally whither away and die at a younger age. All efforts to gain weight failed. But once insulin therapy begins, weight gain and stabilization seems to happen rather quickly.

When we look at type 2 diabetics, we are looking at a population that is already more overweight than the regular population. But ask any medical doctor who has real experience of managing patients up to the point of starting insulin treatment. They will tell you weight gain was likely already taking place, but that it also speeds up significantly upon starting insulin treatment.

Even insulin in non diabetics has the same effect. With the development of an insulinoma, a rare tumor affecting the pancreas that causes persistent insulin release, there is associated weight gain. Once the tumor is removed, we usually see a strong loss in weight thereafter.

Ok, so insulin itself has a clear effect on weight gain. But about things that affect insulin function?

Diabetic medications tell us a lot

Metformin

The first medication commonly prescribed to diabetics to lower blood sugar. Metformin accomplishes this primarily by decreasing the release of glucose from the liver. There are no effects on insulin, and we generally see some weight loss with its treatment. Lower blood sugar means lower insulin.

Alpha glucosidase inhibitors

These medications work by inhibiting some of the absorption of glucose through the digestive tract. Less glucose in the body means less insulin produced. Like metformin, we see some weight loss. Nothing crazy, but what's more important is that we don't see weight gain.

SGLT-2 inhibitors

They do the same thing as above, but act by blocking absorption through the kidneys. Once again; lowered glucose and insulin and we produce weight loss.

Sulfonylurea

Sulfonylureas are a class of medications that work by stimulating insulin secretion from the pancreatic cells. We commonly see weight gain with its use. Not as much as we do with straight insulin use but weight gain nonetheless. More insulin, more weight.

Thiazolidinediones

These medications work by increasing the sensitivity to insulin. This increases the effect of the insulin present in the body. They are not used much anymore. But they did cause weight gain when used.

Plenty of other non-diabetic medications exhibit the same patterns. More insulin or more insulin sensitivity promotes weight gain and vice versa.

Incretin agents

This may be the one exception to the trend we see in medications, and how the effects of insulin validate our overall theory of obesity so far. The flashy new medications Semaglutide and Tirzepatide fall into this category. And while they do increase insulin levels as well as improve insulin sensitivity. They also have a powerful effect on the same part of the hypothalamus that we discussed early; The master weight regulator part of your brain. Anyone who has used them has experienced how powerfully they affect you. Making eating literally difficult at times. This effect seems to override the other smaller effects on insulin.

What can we conclude about insulin now?

It's clear that insulin plays a direct role within the framework of obesity. Insulin is the driver behind the weight set point. It directly acts on the part of the brain that triggers it to then subsequently alter your hunger and metabolism. Elevated insulin levels are directly turning up the thermostat in our bodies, causing slow and steady weight gain. How much you ate and how much exercise impacted your weight loss were merely downstream effects. What about leptin? We know Leptin is the other hormone that also impacts the hypothalamus. It appears to have the opposite effect of insulin. Elevated leptin levels tell your hypothalamus to trigger the opposite effect, promoting the decrease in weight. What we can see so far is that lowering insulin levels, which requires addressing insulin resistance, will subsequently lower leptin levels as well.The relationship between these two hormones is indeed the subject of further needed research.

But why do we see elevated levels of both hormones in obese individuals? There appears to be a sort of resistance that has developed to both hormones. More on how hormone resistance develops later on. The two main hormones that play an integral role in regulating your weight become dysregulated and end up keeping you fat. Because they are not supposed to be chronically elevated when functioning normally. We must lower insulin levels, if we ever expect to win this battle for good.

Why did Atkins and Keto start off well?

Anyone who was paying attention to the diet industry when the Atkins diet started growing in popularity would recall how effective it was at rapid weight loss. People were losing weight, but they were losing weight faster and with what seemed to be less effort than the more traditional approaches. This is a real phenomenon, and it's important to understand because it actually plays an important role in understanding why insulin control is so important for fast loss.

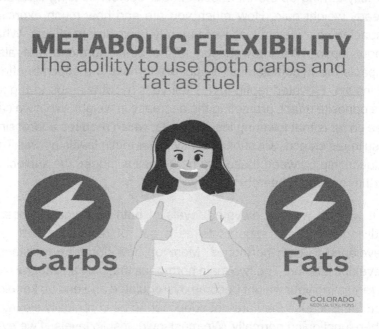

Consuming little to no carbs means there is a much smaller release of insulin after your meals. Fat has almost no effect on insulin release, and protein has a small amount compared to carbs. With much less insulin release, fat mobilization can actually start. This leads to a state of improved metabolic flexibility. This refers to a metabolism's ability to burn both fat and carbs. We will dive into this much deeper in later chapters. But for now, you need to understand that this is the reason Atkins was so successful. It's also the reason the Ketogenic diet is so popular as well. They are essentially the same diet; both consist of consuming a lower number of carbs so that the body is forced to run off fat rather than carbs. The only real difference was that Keto or "Ketogenic" places emphasis on actually entering a state of Ketosis. This is where your body is producing ketone bodies for energy. This was likely happening in people during the Atkins diet era as well, but the program itself did not really mention or emphasize this much. Both scenarios make the body much "better" or more efficient at burning fat. Training fat burning systems, so the metabolism develops "flexibility."

Keep in mind, this is dietary fat that we consume as well as BODY FAT. So it's very logical that weight loss, which is ideally fat loss, would become easier for the body following these approaches. And since it did just that, it was arguably the most popular diet of its time due to its massive success. Ultimately, over time, people began to see the big problem. It's not really sustainable. Don't you think it's really silly to say, "I'm never going to have carbs for the rest of my life." I don't know about you, but there are just too many yummy things that contain carbs. They say sugar is as addictive as cocaine. I think this can be observed In the ravenous carb consumption that would begin for most people who restricted carbs for months or years and then finally take their first bite of carbs. Sadly, many people rebounded and re-gained 30-35% of their weight back within one year.

The keto diet is powerful. And there is an argument to prescribe a keto diet for health reasons such as cancer or neurological cases. But outside these scenarios, it doesn't make sense for everyone else. We need to have a healthy relationship with carbs, and the key to this is moderation when you have built a flexible metabolism.

If you genuinely are happy on a true keto diet and have littler stress living the style, then I'm all for it. I just find that 99.99% of the population wouldn't choose it.

Insulin Resistance

Insulin resistance is a condition in which the body's cells do not respond effectively to the hormone insulin. This leads to impaired glucose uptake, elevated blood sugar levels and excessive weight gain. But how and why does the resistance develop to begin with? Remember earlier where we discussed the massive shift in our diets starting in 1977 and the undeniable appearance of increased rates of obesity right after? It appears that the presence of elevated insulin levels for longer periods of time than what humans were designed to handle has caused a massive adaptive response.

The body operates off a desire to maintain a sort of homeostasis or equilibrium; a balance, really. This is paramount for good survivability. When we walk into a hot building, our bodies cool us off. If we walked into a large freezer, our body would begin to burn calories to produce heat and warm us up. Resistance to a hormone is merely an adaptive response that is trying to return to some healthy balance. Many examples of resistance can be observed

Antibiotics

Antibiotic resistance occurs when bacteria and other microorganisms develop the ability to defeat the drugs designed to kill them; making infections more difficult or even impossible to treat. This is a direct survival mechanism of the bacteria. All living organisms have instinctual survival mechanisms driving them. The ability to become resistant to antibiotics is a result of this. This is a massive concern as it means we could experience a super bug of some sort. A type of infection where no treatment with antibiotics exists. We already saw the first instance of this in 1947. And the possibility of more is very scary. The only real solution so far is to be more cautious when prescribing these medications, but that's a whole other problem entirely.

Exposure over time creates resistance.

Viral Immunity

When it comes to immunity vs. a viral infection, it requires exposure over time as well. When you get the flu, you build a tolerance to it that protects you against future exposure. This is the basis of vaccines as well. The exposure to a weakened version of the virus produces a stronger immune response. AKA resistance created from exposure over time.

Drug resistance

Exposure to drugs over time is no different. Look at anyone who starts to smoke Mary Jane. It doesn't take much to get high. But over time, a tolerance sets in, the user needs to smoke greater and greater amounts to obtain the same effects. Pain medications show us the same resistance at play. And sadly, it ultimately ends up killing millions as the amounts needed to alleviate the pain get so high that the opiates destroy the rest of the body in the process.

Let's look at diabetics again

What is the standard path they head down?

1. They start off with some metformin
2. Then more metformin

3. Then they need 2nd medication
4. Then a 3rd and possibly a 4th.
5. At some point, they have to start injecting some insulin.
6. Then they have to inject more insulin and more insulin.

Remember that big boulder that is rolling uncontrollably down a hill. The more momentum it builds, the harder it would be to stop. Sadly, diabetics are like these boulders, but instead of gravity it's the very treatments themselves pushing them down the hill. We understand that it's the diet primarily that's driving those insulin levels up initially. But there is clearly something else at play beyond this. The diet can only get so crappy up to a point. But we see this continual progression beyond the possibility of the diet still being the primary driver. This is the resistance that has developed at play now. So elevated insulin levels itself over time cause this resistance. However, the only thing the body can do is produce more insulin to get the job done. Remember, insulin's primary job is to get the glucose out of your blood. If it doesn't do this, you would die pretty fast. However, due to the resistance, your body requires more and more insulin.

These poor diabetics are victims of a vicious cycle. The very thing that is keeping them alive is slowly killing them. The continual focus on the management of blood sugar only with more and more medication increasing insulin levels is worsening the resistance and the underlying problem! Let's take a look at other examples of insulin creating insulin resistance.

Although these tumors are rare, insulin producing tumors certainly help to support our working conclusion. Without other diseases present, the person seems to develop insulin resistance in reaction to how much insulin the tumor is producing. If it didn't do this, the person would quickly die from low blood sugar. Another example is Insulin infusions. They have been shown to impair the ability of the body afterward to utilize glucose as effectively, which would demonstrate insulin resistance.

This is a vicious cycle that millions of people are currently stuck in. When you become insulin resistant, it's difficult to climb out. It's no longer just your diet merely driving the weight gain, but now it's the insulin resistance. This is why your efforts to change the diet are not as fruitful anymore. The resistance is the primary reason your insulin levels are high now, and we already understand how insulin keeps us fat. This is the crossing point where it goes from challenging to very hard to lose weight. I think genetics determine how quickly a person develops this resistance, which explains the whole being dealt a crappy hand. Let's finish this hormone journey of ours, so we can get to the solution already.

Cracking the Weight Loss Code: Beyond Calories and Crunches

How does Cortisol come into play

Many experts believe that cortisol management is necessary for successful weight loss. While this can certainly be the case for some people, the effects of cortisol on weight management are simply from its effects on insulin. Cortisol is often referred to as the "stress hormone." It is produced by the adrenal glands and is released in response to stress, helping the body to manage stressors by temporarily pausing regular bodily functions and slowing metabolism. It also increases glucose levels in the blood. Something you would appreciate in a situation where you are running from a tiger.

Unfortunately, this stress response is also triggered by other types of non-physical stress and not just physical dangers. Many people experience daily stressors such as work and family life. These perceived stressors are triggering the same responses. So chronic stressors mean chronically elevated levels of glucose and subsequently elevated levels of insulin. Other negative effects from chronically elevated cortisol levels are:

1. Increased appetite: Elevated cortisol levels can increase appetite and cravings for high-calorie, fatty, and sugary foods. This can lead to overeating and weight gain.
2. Fat storage: Cortisol affects fat distribution by causing fat to be stored centrally, around the organs. Higher long-term cortisol levels are strongly related to having abdominal obesity.
3. Slowed metabolism: Chronic stress and elevated cortisol levels can slow down the metabolism, making it harder for the body to burn calories efficiently

We can see real medical conditions demonstrate this very mechanism at play. Addison's disease is a condition of low levels of cortisol. One classic symptom is lower levels of weight. Cushing syndrome is a condition with high levels of cortisol, and we see the opposite. These people have a hard time losing weight.

What about Thyroid

The thyroid hormone is thought of as the master hormone in our bodies and regulates weight loss. You now understand that thyroid hormone levels are influenced by the hormones insulin and leptin. It's important for clinicians to consider this when properly evaluating the thyroid. Unfortunately, in standard healthcare, the thyroid is poorly managed. This is due to the narrow viewpoint they have regarding the labs. Insurance generally only pays for a single lab called the TSH, which stands for thyroid stimulating hormone.

And while this has some accuracy at predicting the actual status of thyroid levels, it can be wrong in many people. This is why so many people have thyroid symptoms even though their doctor says their thyroid is ok. Or they are on a thyroid prescription, and they still have low thyroid symptoms.

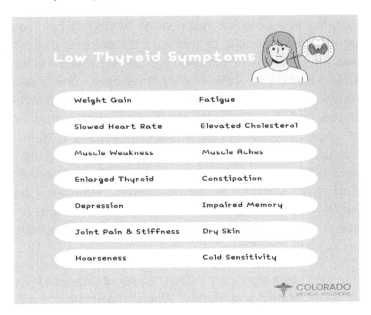

Low Thyroid Symptoms

Weight Gain	Fatigue
Slowed Heart Rate	Elevated Cholesterol
Muscle Weakness	Muscle Aches
Enlarged Thyroid	Constipation
Depression	Impaired Memory
Joint Pain & Stiffness	Dry Skin
Hoarseness	Cold Sensitivity

COLORADO
MEDICAL SOLUTIONS

This is why we do a complete panel with our patients and look at the actual levels of your thyroid levels. If suspect a thyroid issue, then you need to find a clinic/doctor that evaluates at least the following labs in addition to the TSH:

1. Free T3 & T4 – These are free, unbound, actual thyroid hormones that are floating around in your bloodstream.
2. Reverse T3 – This is like a binding protein. It's thought to occupy the T3 receptors to prevent T3 from doing this job. And T3 is the main active thyroid hormone. Somewhere to the tune of 3 to 4 times more active than T4.

If you have an underactive thyroid that fails to respond to a good reset, then there is an augment to be made to optimize with bioidentical thyroid hormone.

I always hear about Inflammation

Inflammation is a biological response to harmful stimuli, such as pathogens, damaged cells, or irritants. It is a complex process that involves the activation of immune cells and the release of various molecules, including inflammatory mediators like cytokines. Cytokines are proteins that regulate immune and inflammatory responses, and some examples of inflammatory mediators include tumor necrosis factor α (TNF-α) and interleukin 6 (IL-6) (22) Inflammation serves to protect the body by eliminating the initial cause of cell injury, clearing out damaged cells and tissues, and initiating the process of tissue repair. However, chronic inflammation can contribute to the development of various chronic conditions, including cardiovascular disease, type 2 diabetes, and certain cancers. (23) (24)

Inflammation has a significant impact on weight loss, as it is closely linked to weight gain and obesity. When inflammation is present, even individuals with disciplined eating and exercise habits may struggle to lose weight.(25) Obesity is associated with chronic inflammation. We know that inflammation also contributes to the development of insulin resistance, leptin resistance, and other metabolic complications. Inflammation increases with weight gain, and reducing inflammation is essential for successful weight loss. (25) Inflammation can also affect the gut microbiota, leading to imbalances that may hinder weight loss efforts. For example, certain gut bacteria may promote inflammation and weight gain, while others may be involved in energy expenditure. (26) (27)

The excess body fat itself stimulates the release of inflammatory mediators such as tumor necrosis factor α and interleukin 6, predisposing the body to a pro-inflammatory state and oxidative stress. (28) (29) This chronic low-grade inflammation, also known as "metaflammation," can contribute to the development of various chronic conditions, including cardiovascular disease, type 2 diabetes, and certain cancers. (30) (31) Inflammation promotes fat gain, and more fat promotes more inflammation. The relationship between inflammation and insulin resistance is also tight. More inflammation will increase the likelihood of developing insulin resistance.

Part Three:
Bridging the Gap: Modern Science & Ancestral Fasting Wisdom

"Fasting is the greatest remedy-- the physician within." — Philippus Paracelsus, one of the three fathers of Western medicine

"Instead of using medicine, better fast today." — Plutarch, a Greek biographer and moralist.

"The best of all medicines is resting and fasting."""—- Benjamin Franklin

"Fasting is considered one of the most ancient healing traditions in the world. The Greek physician, Hippocrates, recommended abstinence from food or drink for patients who exhibited certain symptoms of illness." — Hippocrates

"He who eats until he is sick must fast until he is well."" — English proverb

It's so crazy to think that medical practitioners of the past already knew about how amazing fasting was and how it should be part of the lifestyle. Doctors were known for even prescribing it at times! Unfortunately, over the centuries, that seemed to fade away. And you guys know what happened already after we did the opposite of fasting and started recommending more periodic snacking. It brings me great pleasure to see the emergence of this beautiful lifestyle practice. Unfortunately, it's taking way longer for this beautiful science to emerge and unfortunately millions of people are paying the price with their lives.

Fasting has been around for over a millennium, dating back to the ancient Romans. Many warriors fasted before a big battle. I believe this is because of the brain-boosting effects it provides. Some religions go through some periods of fasting. Some speak of deeper spiritual connection and/or awareness that can be achieved through a fast. While this has not been proven through science, I believe there is something there. What has been proven is strong relaxation and enhanced focus effect induced by positive changes in brain chemistry. More on that later. It would make sense that being in a more relaxed and focused state would better foster the possibility of a spiritual awareness. So let's dive into the science, so we can establish some concrete facts about what fasting can do for you. If you want to take a more in-depth look into the scientific basis of fasting, I suggest you pick up the book: **The Scientific Approach to Intermittent Fasting by Dr. Vanderscheldon.**

The Science of Fasting: A Deeper Dive into Wellness

Before we dive into the science of fasting, I wanted to talk about research in general. I feel people get trapped into this science backed approach that can also be problematic at times. Scientific experiments are the reason we have been able to draw accurate conclusions about the world that we need to advance the way we have and will continue to need as we continue to progress. Unfortunately, the high-level research that helps us draw the most accurate conclusions is very costly. Generally speaking, there has to be money up top that has a clear path to financially gain from spending the millions and sometimes billions of dollars that are necessary to perform the research at that magnitude. The trap that I see many fall into, doctors and non doctors alike, is that they fail to consider this reality. When comparing the efficacy and safety of treatment options for a given condition, for example; there is a tendency to compare research as if there is equal representation existent on both sides. This is far from the case. Because of this, we can get very unfair comparisons in the favor of the side backed by financial interests.

Additionally, there is also a great deal of research bias. Dr. John Loannidis, from Stanford University, is known as being one of the most cited scientists in history. He is well-known for his work on biases in medical research and has published numerous articles on the topic. In 2005, he published a paper titled "Why Most Published Research Findings Are False," which highlighted issues with small study sizes, research bias, competition among scientists, and financial conflicts of interest. He demonstrates how all of this negatively impacts the reliability of "scientific" findings.(1) Dr. Ioannidis is currently the director of the Stanford Prevention Research Center and has also helped launch the Meta-Research Innovation Center at Stanford (METRICS) to improve research accuracy and efficiency across various scientific fields (32).

If we neglect to consider the lack of conclusive research when looking at certain things, as well the great deal of research bias that exists in the high-level research that we do have; then we are left with the path that they want us to take. When looking at lifestyle interventions as long fasting, many still argue that we don't have enough safety studies. While this is a true statement, without considering what's being discussed here, there Millions that could be benefiting now. Conclusive research is important, but given the scene, we need to utilize other things to help us draw conclusions. There is plenty of research that helps us understand the mechanisms at play. Just look at the hormone theory of obesity. If we relied on the highest level research only to conclude it was hormones that are the culprit, it would be a much harder argument to be made. I recommend that if you want the strongest argument for the hormonal theory of obesity that you pick up the book: The Obesity Code by Dr. Jason Fung. Dr. Fung takes all the research that we have and looks at all the mechanisms at play behind obesity and makes a very solid argument as is.

Fasting, in a sense, means going through long periods without eating. I know by now you have likely heard about intermittent fasting or time restricted eating. This is a form of daily fasting that involves taking the window of time in which you eat your calories and narrows that window down to say 10 hours. But you can also do the extreme version, which is one meal per day and usually that would take about an hour or so and then you would fast for the other 23 hours of the day. While I love the longer fasting methods, I'm not as much of a fan of this one, and I'll discuss it in more detail in the appendix. As you know by now, my favorite form of fasting is prolonged fasting. There Is no technical definition of this style of fasting. This is part of the reason I created the FLOA protocol. Fasting becomes much less understood and less discussed once you get beyond the intermittent realm. But most sources say once you pass 24 to 36 hours that you enter the prolonged fasting area, and I 100% agree with this. Simply put, the benefits of prolonged fasting compared to intermittent fasting are night and day. All the benefits you get from intermittent are enhanced. You also experience many new benefits when tapping into this awesomeness. My goal for you by the end of this section is to understand how silly it is that you haven't already been implementing this easy to do lifestyle hack. And for you to be excited to start your long fasting with me on your journey back to a better you.

The human body is truly wonderful. If left with just water, most people would survive for a lot longer than you would think. In fact…

"Altogether, it seems possible to survive without food and drink within a time span of 8 to 21 days. If a person is only deprived of food, the survival time may even go up to about two months, although this is influenced by many factors." (178)

In general, it is likely that a person could survive between 1 and 2 months without food.It makes a lot of sense if you think of our ancestors. They literally had no choice but to be able to survive days, and at times likely weeks without eating. Every meal was a literal job to acquire. Millions of years of evolution and survival of the fittest produced the genetic material that we are all a result of today. Literally, In your body, you have the genes of the people who evolved to develop the best capabilities of handling a variable schedule of eating. Additionally, if bodies grew weak during times of famine, their likelihood of a successful hunt would be poor. Humans have only lived in societies with a more steady supply of food for approximately 10,000 years, since the Neolithic Revolution. This period marked a significant shift in human history, as people transitioned from being hunter-gatherers to farmers. The development of agriculture allowed for a more stable and reliable food supply, which in turn led to the growth of human populations and the formation of complex societies.(33) Compare this short length of time to how long humans have existed: 3 million years ago (34).

It's no different in the animal kingdom, either. Many animals eat a large meal and then go days or weeks before the next one. The human body has a large amount of energy stores in the form of fat. The average 200 lb male at 25% body fat would have 50 lbs of fat on their body. Let's only access 20lbs of that fat. There are 3500 calories in a single pound of body fat. The average daily metabolic rate of a man of this size at rest would be 2500 calories, give or take some. It would take 28 days to burn through 20 pounds of body fat if they consumed zero calories and performed no exercise. Additionally, the body would go into starvation mode much sooner than 28 days of no food and slow down the metabolic rate in an effort to stay alive. So it would actually take longer than 28 days to lose 20 lbs. The human body was built too fast, it has evolved to survive periods of time with no food quite effectively. By not regularly performing periods of fasting that are at least 36 hours or more but less than 96 hours, we are missing one critical pillar of health. But more importantly, we are missing the boat on what I believe to be the most powerfully effective strategy for healthy weight loss attainment and maintenance.

I love using ancestral wisdom as I wage my war with obesity by providing this easy to follow FLOA protocol. Earlier, we learned all about the hormone insulin. It should be easier now to understand why it's all about LOWERING INSULIN. Hands down, this is it. This trumps everything else bar none. It is my strong opinion that regularly fasting for longer periods is the best approach towards lowering insulin levels. This is why the Atkins/keto diets were so successful because they initially produced the same benefits. They crushed the insulin levels. Remember that insulin resistance develops from persistent insulin levels over time. The literal opposite of that would be low levels of insulin over time; something Atkins, keto and fasting all provide. It's this scenario that allows for healing from the insulin resistance. But we cannot forget reality and the importance of finding a practical lifestyle that most would agree sounds much more realistic to maintain. Committing to never having a piece of bread for the rest of your life is pretty silly. Fasting really is the answer.

For many, though, intermittent fasting is simply not enough. It wasn't for me, and I have worked with patients for over a decade now, seeing the same thing in many of them. But prolonged fasting is usually enough for most if it's done consistently enough. This is what led me to create the FLOA protocol. The FLOA protocol is a structured approach towards prolonged fasting. The main objectives of FLOA are:

1. Restoring healthy weight and normalizing metabolic function.
2. Maintaining a healthy weight with ease due to the normalization of metabolic health.

Healing Insulin Resistance

Fasting lowers insulin levels simply by removing the need for your body to produce insulin to begin with. We understand that the presence of insulin in the bloodstream directly prevents fat oxidation. Doesn't mean you can't lose weight, but the percentage of that weight coming from fat is severely reduced. It also allows for the healing of the insulin receptor sites. Your body is a genius design, and it wants to heal everything back to the most optimal it can be, and will take it as far as it can at all times. The resistance to insulin was a physiological adaptation it felt was in your favor due to always having chronically elevated insulin levels. Over a long enough period of time of lowering insulin levels via prolonged fasting, the insulin resistance improves. (35) The improvement of insulin resistance leads to the overall chronically elevated levels of insulin starting to drop. Remember, the two main things driving your insulin levels up were your diet and the resistance itself.

This sets off a cascade of downstream events in the body necessary to start weight loss:

1. Fat to be burned for fuel.
2. Improvement in leptin resistance causes the body to begin to respond to leptin, which is trying to tell you the entire time how much extra fat it needs to burn off, and to make it happen by changing your metabolic rate and hunger levels.

3. Better energy delivery to where the body needs it, thus decreasing the demand for it. That demand was hunger, so now you have less of it.
4. Reduction in inflammation

Inflammation

The 2nd most important variable we need to handle is inflammation. You learned earlier about how it affects weight loss. The reason that it is number two for me is that I have found, in my clinical experience, that the insulin issue is a more common issue for most people than inflammation is. But make no mistake, inflammation can derail you as well. So how does fasting reduce inflammation?

First, let's look at the magical biological process that takes place when you get into a deep fast called cellular autophagy. This is a process in which the body consumes itself. Sounds like something out of an old science fiction horror film. But it really is a wonderful process, I promise. The cells in our body are considered the smallest form of life. They contain their own "cellular organs," like organs of the human body, called organelles. These organelles grow older as the cells age and affect the overall performance of each cell. We have trillions of cells in the body, and it can said that the overall level of vitality of a person at any moment is the average overall health status of each cell.(36) (37) It's impossible to be at 100% because various cells are on a certain timeline towards cellular death. When the process of autophagy is activated from fasting, your body begins to clean the house. It begins to break down these lower functioning organelles and recycle them for amino acids to be used for more essential cells in the body, such as the brain and heart tissues. When you come out of the fasted state and consume calories again, the body is now signaled to rebuild brand-new organelles and cells that fell victim to this cellular consuming process known as cellular autophagy. This process will lower your inflammation along the way. (38)

Other things that fasting does to reduce inflammation

1. It can "turn off" some of the inflammatory pathways or reset them to stop the inflammatory cascade.
2. It can "turn off" inflammatory cytokines and immune cells and "calms down" the angry inflammation-producing cells.
3. Improve circulating glucose and lipid levels
4. Fasting can reduce the number of pro-inflammatory cells called monocytes in the blood.
5. Fasting can reduce the production of free radicals, which can cause inflammation

Metabolic flexibility

We are going to discuss the many benefits of fasting. But I want you to remember three specifically, as they are the ones that are most important to your issue with healthy and easy weight management. Insulin, inflammation, and metabolic flexibility. We learned all about metabolic flexibility earlier, and it's part of why Keto/Atkins diets start off so successfully. This ability to be very metabolically flexible is part of the equation in how our patients can easily maintain their weight after our program. We call this the FLOA lifestyle, more on this later. This is an even bigger deal for people using the flashy new GLP-1 medications to starve themselves skinny. More on this later as well.

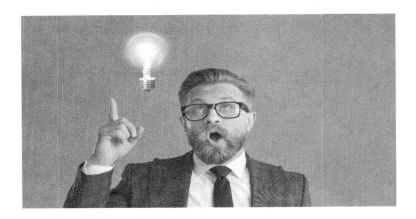

The regular rounds of long fasting are what got the changes needed, and it's also what is going to allow us to maintain it for the rest of our lives. The main difference being that you won't need to fast as frequently in the future to maintain your weight. Fasting for long periods of time may still sound like an impossible feat, and I thoroughly understand. We haven't discussed the "Modern Science " part of this section title yet ☺ But just pretend for now I made it easy. I think the testimonials and great deal of popularity over our program speaks for itself. So diving into prolonged fasting is made easy with some science backed help. As you do the FLOA protocol more and more, you become more and more metabolically flexible. The more flexible you become, the easier it is for your body to FLOA fast. Making it easier for you means you won't need as much of that science – backed help that we are going to discuss soon. You see where I'm going with this??

Let's dive into the other amazing health benefits of fasting.

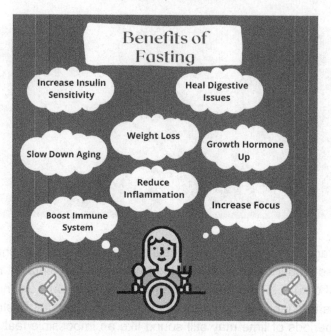

Calorie smashing

Calorie smashing is one of those benefits that always strums an "oh yea" sort of response when one really begins to understand it. What do I mean by "calorie smashing?" What I'm referring to is taking advantage of a much easier way to create a large calorie deficit. To lose weight, we must consume fewer calories than we burn. While we have learned that it is your hormones driving your hunger and metabolic rate, you can still consciously or emotionally override this. There is no diet where you can consume more calories over a period of time than what you burn and still lose weight in that period of time. It's just not possible. So, whatever you are doing to lose weight, there has to be some sort of caloric deficit over time. Meaning, at the end of each period of time, we burn more than they consume. The problem with this is not only the difficulty itself of maintaining a caloric deficit day in and day out, but the effect on the metabolism over a prolonged period of doing so. Eventually, your body reacts by slowing down your metabolic rate. You understand the science of this already. In the fitness world, we have always called this a weight loss plateau. When in a metabolic plateau, you may notice some of the low thyroid symptoms such as constipation, intolerance to cold, lower levels of energy and brain fog. It's a scary place to be, for sure. You are exercising a lot, eating less and no longer dropping weight. Many people get frustrated and less motivated. This leads to less effort on the exercise and diet front, and this leads to rebound weight. They begin to gain weight with much less effort than before the weight loss ever started. This is because they are literally now burning fewer calories at rest than what they were burning before. So this sort of approach is not only difficult in of itself, but it also leads to a plateau for many people.

So the plateau is awful, and calorie restriction overtime causes this. How do we keep smashing calories and burning lots of fat with less effort but also avoid it? By ensuring you eat at your TEE on the five days. Even being over this each day is totally acceptable due to how massive the calorie deficit is from the 48-hour fast. Your metabolism is much less likely to go into starvation mode when done in this manner. Calorie restriction, over time, creates the plateau. This is strategy at its best. This is playing to the design of the body. It would appear the body doesn't detect this scenario the same as it does with a consistent calorie restriction. We will get into the implementation of this program in later chapters. But for now, you can get excited that this is real and many of our patients can attest to this.

Scan here to see Testimonials:

Let's look at the numbers, so you can better see the strategy here. Remember, the average person burns 2000 calories at rest per day and there are 3500 calories in a pound of body fat. So, if you are fasting for 48 hours per week, in theory you will lose 1-2 lbs. of fat with NO EXERCISE. Actually, the scale will show about 3 to 5 lbs of loss for most people due to water weight loss. Carbs are stored in the body with water, so when you fast for 48 hours you deplete your stored carbs, so you lose a lot of water weight as well. This is why we have our patients weigh themselves once per week on the day before the long fast so that we can account for the weekly water weight loss and regain. Back to the calories. So saying 2000 calories at rest, that's a 4000 calorie deficit we just created!!!! Now let's compare the effort to obtain this in a diet/exercise program. An average jogger burns 500 calories per hour. Let's say they are doing 4 hours per week. That is about 2000 calories. Additionally, they are eating about 300 calories less per day, so that's also about

2000 calories. So that also comes out to the same net loss of fat. Even ignoring the fact that this approach will lead to a starvation mode response in a variable amount of time, person to person; which scenario looks better to you? Let me remind you that the other 5 days of eating require you to eat a full day of food. No caloric deficit these days are allowed. Which scenario is more sustainable?

Powerful effects on muscle perseveration and growth

Fasting can have positive effects on muscle preservation during weight loss through hormonal optimization. When fasting, the body experiences several hormonal changes, such as a decrease in insulin and leptin levels and an increase in growth hormone levels (39) There is also an increase in "flight or fight" hormones called catecholamines. Finally, the production of ketone bodies as it shifts its fuel source towards fat and away from carbs is also helpful with protecting muscle mass.

Growth hormone(GH) plays major roles in muscle development. It influences muscle growth through various mechanisms, including the regulation of insulin-like growth factor 1 (IGF-1), which is a potent regulator of muscle mass in health and disease. GH can increase protein synthesis in muscle cells, as demonstrated in a study on bovine skeletal muscle cells, where GH increased protein synthesis in myotubes (muscle fibers formed by the fusion of myoblasts.) It can literally increase the number of muscle fibers you have.(40) Not even anabolic steroids can do this.

Increased catecholamine production influences muscle mass by affecting various cellular processes. For example, activation of the adrenergic receptor has a positive impact on muscle mass (41). It can also stimulate muscle growth by increasing protein synthesis and regulating the expression of muscle growth-related genes (2). Think adrenaline here. They give you a heightened sense of awareness and help you deal with stress. Allowing muscle breakdown during this period of lack of food is the opposite of handling the stress of needing to kill your next meal.

Ketone bodies have been shown to be very anti-catabolic. These hormonal changes can contribute to a shift from glucose to lipid oxidation, which may help preserve muscle mass during weight loss. (39) Ketone bodies play a role in preserving muscle mass by influencing energy metabolism and reducing muscle protein breakdown. A study looked at various cellular influences by ketone bodies and demonstrated anti-catabolic impact on muscle protein. (42)

In a study on the effects of prolonged fasting on various components within skeletal muscle from lean and obese individuals, it was found that fasting led to a decrease in plasma insulin and leptin levels and an increase in growth hormone levels in both lean and obese subjects (43). This suggests that fasting-induced hormonal changes can impact muscle preservation in individuals with different body compositions. Ketone production during fasting periods of less than 4 days can have an impact on muscle mass preservation. When fasting, the body shifts from using glucose to ketone bodies as its primary fuel source. This shift can help conserve muscle mass, as gluconeogenesis from amino acids is reduced when ketone bodies become the major fuel source (44)

We do understand that fasting beyond this 4 to 5-day period is where we start to see muscle wasting. This again makes a lot of evolutionary sense. Muscle is a more metabolically active tissue than fat mass. It requires more calories at rest to exist. After five days, the body is now thinking "I need to slow down the metabolism as much as possible" for maximal survival.

Mood and Motivation

Prolonged fasting can have several positive effects on mood and motivation. Some of these positive effects include:

1. Enhanced mental clarity: During fasting, the body shifts its energy source from glucose to ketone bodies, which can provide a more efficient fuel source for the brain. This shift can lead to improved mental clarity and focus, which may positively impact mood and motivation.(45).
2. Increased production of brain-derived neurotrophic factor (BDNF): Fasting has been shown to increase the production of BDNF, a protein that supports the growth and maintenance of neurons in the brain. Higher levels of BDNF have been associated with improved mood, reduced anxiety, and increased resilience to stress.(45)
3. Reduced inflammation: Prolonged fasting can help reduce inflammation in the body, which has been linked to various mood disorders, such as depression and anxiety. (46) By reducing inflammation, fasting may help improve mood and overall mental well-being.
4. Autophagy and cellular repair: Fasting can stimulate autophagy, a process by which the body cleans out damaged cells and regenerates new, healthy ones. (179) This cellular repair process may contribute to improved mood and motivation by promoting overall brain health.
5. Hormonal balance: Fasting can help regulate hormone levels, such as cortisol and insulin, which can have a positive impact on mood and motivation. (180) Balanced

hormone levels can lead to increased energy, improved sleep, and reduced stress

Prolonged fasting can influence dopamine levels and motivation. Dopamine is a neurotransmitter that plays a crucial role in reward and motivation, and its levels can be affected by various factors, including fasting. During fasting, the body undergoes several hormonal and metabolic changes that can impact dopamine neurotransmission (47)

In a study on the effects of fasting on dopamine neurotransmission in the brain of male and female mice, it was found that fasting promotes dopamine release and reuptake in these regions, which is involved in motivation and reward (181). This suggests that fasting may enhance motivation by modulating dopamine levels in specific brain regions

Another study on the effects of fasting during Ramadan found that participants experienced significantly less fatigue and improvements in mood-related symptoms after they began fasting compared to before fasting (48). This improvement in mood and motivation could be related to changes in dopamine levels during fasting

Blood sugar management

Another huge health benefit of fasting is blood sugar regulation. Diabetes is a huge epidemic and a horrible disease to deal with. Prediabetes and type 2 diabetes are conditions in which the body responds less to the insulin that it makes. Therefore, as a side effect, the blood sugar rises. Once it gets high enough, your doctor begins to put you on various medications to control your blood sugar. These medications do little for the real problem, insulin resistance. They merely keep your blood sugar from damaging your body and ultimately killing you. Over time, they usually need to change your medications to stronger cocktails of medications because the insulin resistance continues to get worse. For many patients, they hit a point where they become insulin-dependent type 2 Diabetics. The medications are no longer strong enough, so they must inject insulin. Guess what? This only perpetuates the issue. Who would have thought that blasting your cells with a much larger dose of insulin than your pancreas would ever produce in one moment would only desensitize your cells even more? Aka, make the insulin resistance get worse

The only way to get out of this worsening situation is to re-sensitize the cells in your body or combat the insulin resistance. This is accomplished through lifestyle interventions. And wouldn't you have guessed it.... Prolonged fasting is freaking fantastic at doing just that.

SIDE NOTE: For the diabetics reading this that are very insulin resistant, utilizing this therapy first to help reverse your insulin resistance to a point where you can then tap into the wonderful benefits of prolonged fasting makes a lot of sense.

Scan the QR Code for more information on this therapy.

One of my favorite perks of fasting is the time savings it affords you. It also eliminates the excuse of not having enough time to lose weight. You literally don't have to exercise for this to work, and spend much time worrying about food preparation and the act of eating itself. By the way, we are not advocating to not exercise. But we have many patients who come to us in poor health. They couldn't exercise even if they wanted too due to pain and various conditions. We also get many patients with extremely busy lifestyles who cannot add 5 days of exercise to their schedule. Exercise is incredible and there are a plethora of books to read about, but my point here is that if you truly have a schedule that doesn't allow for the number of workouts that you would have needed to do to lose weight in the past or if your body won't allow you to do so…. Well, now you won't need to stress about that, and you will still likely lose weight. I promise.

Cancer prevention

Prolonged fasting has been suggested to have potential cancer prevention benefits, mainly based on preclinical studies. Some of the mechanisms through which prolonged fasting may contribute to cancer prevention include:

1. Reduced inflammation: Prolonged fasting can help reduce inflammation in the body, which has been linked to various types of cancer (49).
2. Enhanced autophagy: Fasting can stimulate autophagy, a process by which the body cleans out damaged cells and regenerates new, healthy ones. This cellular repair process may contribute to cancer prevention by promoting overall cellular health (182).
3. Hormonal balance: Fasting can help regulate hormone levels, such as insulin and insulin-like growth factor 1 (IGF-1), which have been associated with cancer development and progression (50)

Cancer development and progression usually involves and an overactive and dysregulated mTOR signaling. The mTOR pathway plays a crucial role in regulating various cellular functions, including cell growth, proliferation, survival, and metabolism(1). Dysregulation of the mTOR pathway is frequently reported in many types of human tumors, and targeting this pathway has been considered an attractive potential therapeutic target in cancer (51)

During fasting, the mTOR pathway can be inhibited, leading to an increase in autophagy, a process by which the body cleans out damaged cells and regenerates new, healthy ones (52). Inhibition of the mTOR pathway during fasting can also lead to changes in various signaling pathways that can impact cellular processes,

95

such as protein synthesis and degradation, which may have implications for overall health and disease prevention. (52)

Cancer is a process of abnormal, excessive growth. This is why a growth hormone increase from various peptide therapies available, is not a good thing for people with cancer. Fasting is an anti-growth process. It's a good contrast to balance out the growth that a good deal of health optimization enthusiasts are looking to take advantage of.

Heart health

Fasting can improve heart health through various mechanisms, including:

1. Reduced inflammation: Prolonged fasting can help reduce inflammation in the body, which has been linked to various types of heart diseases (53).
2. Improved lipid profile: Fasting has been shown to positively affect lipid profiles, such as reducing total cholesterol and LDL cholesterol levels, and increasing HDL cholesterol levels. These changes can contribute to a reduced risk of cardiovascular diseases (54).
3. Weight loss: Fasting can promote weight loss, which can help improve heart health by reducing the strain on the heart and decreasing the risk of developing obesity-related heart diseases (54.)
4. Blood pressure regulation: Fasting has been associated with improvements in blood pressure regulation, which can help reduce the risk of hypertension and related heart diseases (55.)

96

5. Improved insulin sensitivity: Fasting can improve insulin sensitivity, which can help prevent or manage type 2 diabetes, a risk factor for heart diseases (54).

Enhanced brain function

Fasting can improve overall brain function and help prevent neurodegenerative diseases through various mechanisms:

1. Enhanced autophagy: Fasting stimulates autophagy, a process by which the body cleans out damaged cells and regenerates new, healthy ones. This cellular repair process may contribute to improved brain health and reduced risk of neurodegenerative diseases (183).
2. Increased production of brain-derived neurotrophic factor (BDNF): Fasting has been shown to increase the production of BDNF, a protein that supports the growth and maintenance of neurons in the brain. Higher levels of BDNF have been associated with improved cognitive function and reduced risk of neurodegenerative diseases, such as Alzheimer's and Parkinson's disease (56.)
3. Reduced inflammation: Prolonged fasting can help reduce inflammation in the body, which has been linked to various neurodegenerative diseases (57)
4. Improved insulin sensitivity: Fasting can improve insulin sensitivity, which can help prevent or manage type 2 diabetes, a risk factor for neurodegenerative diseases (56).
5. Regulation of mTOR pathway: Fasting can inhibit the mTOR pathway, which plays a crucial role in regulating various cellular functions, including cell growth, cell division, survival, and metabolism. Dysregulation of the mTOR pathway is frequently reported in many types of human tumors, and targeting the signaling pathway has been

considered an attractive potential therapeutic target in cancer (58.)

In the context of specific neurodegenerative diseases, studies have shown benefits of intermittent fasting for Alzheimer's disease and multiple sclerosis on disease symptoms and progress (59). Animal studies also suggest that Parkinson's disease, autism spectrum disorder, and mood and anxiety disorders could benefit from intermittent fasting (56).

Anti-aging and longevity

Fasting can improve overall anti-aging and longevity through various mechanisms:

1. Enhanced autophagy: Fasting stimulates autophagy, a process by which the body cleans out damaged cells and regenerates new, healthy ones. This cellular repair process may contribute to improved overall health and reduced risk of age-related diseases (60.)
2. Regulation of nutrient-sensing pathways: Fasting can affect nutrient-sensing pathways, such as the mTOR pathway, which plays a crucial role in regulating various cellular functions, including cell growth, proliferation, survival, and metabolism. Inhibition of the mTOR pathway during fasting can lead to increased autophagy and potential health benefits (61.)
3. Reduced inflammation: Prolonged fasting can help reduce inflammation in the body, which has been linked to various age-related diseases (62.)
4. Improved insulin sensitivity: Fasting can improve insulin sensitivity, which can help prevent or manage type 2 diabetes, a risk factor for age-related diseases (61).

98

5. Increased production of ketone bodies: Fasting can lead to the production of ketone bodies, which have been shown to have anti-aging effects by activating specific receptors and contributing to the anti-vascular aging effect of autophagy (63).

6. Hormonal balance: Fasting can help regulate hormone levels, such as insulin and insulin-like growth factor 1 (IGF-1), which have been implicated in the aging process (61)

It is important to note that individual experiences with fasting may vary, and the positive effects on anti-aging and longevity can be influenced by factors such as metabolic responses, duration of fasting, and overall health. However, many people report experiencing improved overall health and reduced signs of aging during and after prolonged fasting periods (62)

The Best Stimulus for Healthy Cellular Autophagy

Fasting triggers autophagy, a cellular process that helps maintain cellular health and homeostasis by degrading and recycling damaged cellular components, such as proteins and organelles (63). Autophagy is activated during fasting as a response to nutrient deprivation, which allows cells to recycle their components and generate energy to maintain essential cellular functions (63). Here are some key aspects of how fasting triggers autophagy:

1. Nutrient sensing pathways: Fasting affects nutrient-sensing pathways, such as the mTOR pathway, which plays a crucial role in regulating various cellular functions, including cell growth, proliferation, survival, and metabolism (64). Inhibition of the mTOR pathway during fasting can lead to increased autophagy (65).

99

2. Hormonal regulation: Fasting can help regulate hormone levels, such as insulin and insulin-like growth factor 1 (IGF-1), which have been implicated in the activation of autophagy (66).

3. Cellular stress response: Fasting can induce cellular stress, which can activate autophagy as a protective mechanism to maintain cellular homeostasis and promote cell survival (67).

4. Energy conservation: During fasting, cells need to conserve energy and resources. Autophagy allows cells to recycle damaged or unnecessary components, providing energy and building blocks for essential cellular processes (68)

Safety

So we can see how badass fasting is. And we can understand how the longer fasting would produce even more positive changes. But how safe is it? A study on the effects of prolonged fasting in adults with type 1 diabetes found that a 7-day fast was feasible, beneficial, and safe when conducted under medical supervision (69). The study reported no significant adverse events related to fasting, and participants experienced improvements in blood glucose control and insulin requirements. Another study investigated the safety of a 10-day fasting regimen in a hospital-based setting, comparing the efficacy and safety of lower limb orthopedic surgeries (70). The study found no significant differences in complications between the two groups, suggesting that prolonged fasting can be safe when conducted under medical supervision

Some of the strongest studies on the safety of fasting include:

1. A systematic review and meta-analysis on the clinical effect and safety of new preoperative fasting time guidelines for

elective surgery. This study compared the new guidelines put forward by the American Association of Anesthesiologists (fasting for 6 hours, no drinking for 2 hours) with traditional protocols (fasting for 8-12 hours and no drinking for 4-6 hours). The study found that the new guidelines were safe and effective for elective surgery (71).

2. A systematic review and meta-analysis on the safety assessment of glucose-lowering drugs and the importance of structured education during Ramadan fasting. This study found that healthcare professionals play a pivotal role in managing diabetes-related complications in patients who fast during Ramadan, and that there is a need for standard guidelines and structured education in association with drug administration and dosage (72)

Maintaining weight for life aka the FLOA lifestyle

The most important variable for effectively maintaining weight loss is preventing insulin resistance again. The secret to the FLOA lifestyle is less frequent rounds of the same style of FLOA fasting. The magic is in those 36-72 hour time ranges. Even if your diet started to slip up, how the heck could your cells ever become resistant to insulin again when they are given these routine breaks? Remember, insulin resistance is a product of: *Elevated insulin levels over time*

I do believe you would have to try really hard to become resistant again with this routine in place along the daily intermittent fasting. More on the FLOA lifestyle protocols later.

While calories matter significantly less than once thought; they will matter somewhat. So let's look at two scenarios here; A and B. You are eating the same number of weekly calories and maintaining weight in both scenarios. Let's say it takes 10,000 calories each week to maintain your weight for simple numbers here. In A, you are eating 1/7th of 10,000 or about 1428 calories per day. In B you are fasting one of the days entirely. So you are eating about 1667 calories per day during the rest of the week. In scenario B you are cleansing your body each week and giving it time to perform a very healthy biological process. More importantly, albeit the reason you are reading this book, in B, you eat more every single non fasting day. How much easier do you think it is to maintain your weight when you literally have to eat more just to break even in calorie requirements?

Let's summarize it all

Here's the bullet point summary of science backed benefits of fasting. And as a reminder, prolonged fasting enhances these results. And as another reminder; the FLOA protocol is the world's more aggressive format of prolonged fasting.

1. Heals insulin resistance and helps maintain lower levels over time.
2. Reduces inflammation through various mechanisms.
3. Establishes metabolic flexibility, turning us into fast burning machines.
4. Gives you a lot more flexibility in your meal sizes, which fosters a healthy social life.
5. Promotes a more muscular physique via hormonal optimization.
6. Improves your mood and motivation by optimizing brain chemistry.
7. Stabilizes blood sugar levels.

8. Plays vital roles in cancer prevention by acting to inhibit one of the main overactive pathways in cancer progression: mTOR.
9. Improves heart health.
10. Enhances brain function and protects against neurodegenerative diseases like Alzheimer's.
11. It is the most powerful and lowest cost form of anti-aging and longevity.
12. It is the most powerful stimulator of life sustaining cellular autophagy.
13. Plenty of high level safety studies to address our concerns.
14. It is essential for easier weight and health management.

The two major roadblocks most people would bring up when asked to consider a 48-hour fast are hunger and energy levels. One of my favorite parts of the initial weight loss consultation is explaining to the potential patient that we are going to put them on a 48-hour fast. I'm usually met with a wide-eyed look. But in the majority of conversations I have had with patients over the years, I have learned a few things. While many think this idea is impossible, very few ever tried anything remotely close to a 48-hour fast! So the stress level over how hard they think it is begins to subside as I explain how it all works. Now let's talk about the trendy new powerhouse drugs in the weight loss arena. But we won't stop there. Let's discuss many scientifically backed forms of making this easier for you to start.

The World's Most Powerful Appetite Suppressant Compounds

Now, here's the part where we can use some science to hack our way into making this as easy as humanly possible. The GLP-1 medications, Semaglutide and Tirzepatide, are the most powerful options available to aid in your FLOA protocol journey. More on our program differences later.

For more information on our coaching programs or if you simply want to access to FLOA university to help better earn implement all aspects of the FLOA protocol scan the QR Code below:

These medications are known as GLP-1s in slang because they act on the Glucagon-Like Peptide receptors. The first one to go viral and still going hard is known as Semaglutide, which is the active ingredient in Ozempic; the pharmaceutical name for a diabetes medication. They have since approved and released Wegovy which has the same active ingredient as Ozempic, Semaglutide, but is approved specifically for obesity. There has since been a more powerful medication released known as Tirzepatide, which is the active ingredient in Mounjaro, the pharmaceutical name for another diabetic medication. We will also discuss Retratrutide, the latest drug not yet approved for anything yet at the time of writing this book.

These medications are a remarkable aid to battling hunger and cravings. They shut down that "food noise" that roadblocks most people from starting some lifestyle improvements that involve eating less food and less junk food. Originally, they were made for type 2 diabetes treatment by controlling blood sugar levels, but they were also found to have this powerful hunger-controlling side effect. This is simply due to the mechanism of action of GLP-1 receptor stimulation. These compounds exist naturally in our bodies; they are referred to as incretin hormones. They are released in response to eating, to tell us that we are full and to make us stop eating. These medications are modified versions of these naturally occurring peptide hormones to be significantly more powerful. Jiminy jillikers batman! These things are magic. The level of appetite suppression is out of this world. Many things have been marketed and touted as appetite suppressing. But they all pale in comparison to the effect of these medications. To give you some comparison, if you are familiar with it, it suppresses your appetite even more powerfully than Phentermine or "Fen-Phen." But most importantly, it's an entirely different class of compound. It's not a stimulant at all, so it doesn't have all the nasty side effects such as spiking blood pressure that makes medications like Fen-Phen much less favorable.

If you look deeper into the mechanism of action of these GLP1 medications, you see that they improve insulin secretion. This may be a bit confusing to comprehend if you paid any attention to what we taught you about insulin's effect on your weight. The massive appetite-suppressing effects appear to override the increase in insulin they provide. Remember that the way insulin keeps you from weight loss is its effect on the brain, which then in turn increases your appetite. This drug seems to bypass insulin's normal effect and triggers the same part of the brain to induce massive appetite suppression. This also makes sense when you consider the rapid rebound weight gain after stopping the medication. Insulin gets back to doing its things after the drug leaves the body, and presto; fast weight gain begins. This is one of the many reasons I advocate short-term use, if you will be using it at all. We will dive into all this later on.

Let's distinguish between purchasing the pharmaceutical versions vs. other products. In the case of using Semaglutide, you are using the active ingredient that is in Ozempic and Wegovy. But you are not using the same product as the pharmaceutical companies. The pharmaceutical companies have not provided their formulas to the public, as it is their intellectual property. Semaglutide can also be compounded at state-licensed compounding pharmacies. There was a natural shortage of these medications, and when that happens to any medication, the FDA allows state licensed compounding pharmacies to compound the medications themselves. These pharmacies are not regulated by the FDA. State pharmacy boards instead regulate them. The standards for safety and efficacy are still very high in order for these pharmacies to remain compliant.

Unfortunately, there are other sources that people can find these medications. There exist online companies that refer to themselves as "research companies." These companies can legally sell all sorts of drugs and peptides by labeling them for "research only" and "not for human consumption." It's a bit of a joke, though; everyone familiar with these operations knows they are being used for human consumption. What concerns me the most is the lack of safety standards for these so-called "labs." They can tell people whatever the hell they want to make the sale. They can show you all the safety and efficacy "studies." But there is zero regulatory agency there to enforce anything on them. It blows my mind how trusting people can be when injecting things into their body

Using medications such as Ozempic or Mounjaro can give some certainty to the user that you are getting what they paid for. However, you are paying a very high premium for this certainty. The pharmaceutical companies have started protecting their interests by filing lawsuits against companies advertising products like Semaglutide and presenting them as pharmaceutical versions. I respect their decisions to protect their interest as they spent the money to get the clinical trials done. What I don't appreciate are the scare tactics that I see drawing concerns about any product containing the same active ingredients that are not the pharmaceutical version. I agree, everyone should run like hell from the research companies. But products coming from compounding pharmacies can be a real viable option. They are significantly cheaper than the pharmaceutical versions. I have personally visited the labs of the pharmacies we work with and feel very comfortable with the standards they uphold. We let all of our patients know they are not getting Ozempic or Mounjaro, for example, if they are getting Tirzepatide from us.

Furthermore, I think it's essential to clarify the idea of "taking away from diabetics." Yes, there is a natural shortage, as explained, and this is why the FDA allowed compounding pharmacies to begin production. These versions do not replace the versions that insurance companies would cover for people with diabetes. Insurance would not cover these versions. The idea, though, is that there will be less off-label usage of the insurance covered medications due to people using these compounded products instead. This would free up the supply for diabetics. So please don't let an uneducated person tell you otherwise.

Let's take a brief dive into the differences between these products.

Semaglutide, aka Ozempic or Wegovy

Ozempic, was approved by the FDA in 2017 for treating diabetes. But due to how damn effective it is for weight loss and the celebrity endorsement because of this; its off-label usage skyrocketed and likely had lots to do with the natural shortage.

The research is unequivocal in its effectiveness.

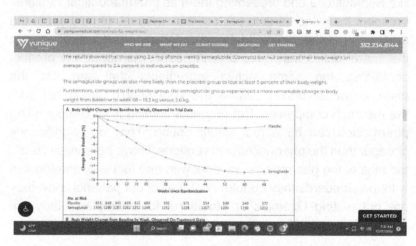

Participants lost an average of about .5% of their body weight each week. This is tangible evidence that Semaglutide works. But if I'm being honest, the results pale in comparison to what we have been seeing with our patients. Usually, our program has been yielding closer to 1-1.5% of weight loss per week.

(You can see TESTIMONIALS here.)

Tirzepatide, aka Mounjaro

Mounjaro was FDA approved for the treatment of diabetes in May 2022. It is not yet approved for Obesity, but that is likely to happen late 2023 or early 2024. What's special about Tirzepatide is its dual mechanism of action. It not only works on the GLP-1 receptors, but it also acts on the GIP receptors as well. In a nutshell, the literature has shown that Tirzepatide outperforms Semaglutide in all categories and even has a lower side effect profile. Tirzepatide is our GLP-1 of choice because of this. I have personally witnessed and experienced the difference between them both.

Retatrutide

The soon-to-be new kid on the block is Retatrutide. Preliminary research indicates that it's even more effective than Tirzepatide. It just passed phase two clinical trials. This medication has a triple mechanism of action that adds even more potential effect than Tirzepatide. I don't see it being of that much interest for us, though. It does happen at times with the very inflamed, obese and/or insulin resistant needing more appetite suppression to break the initial barriers, but it's rare.

Other Worthy Mentions of Medication-based Appetite Suppression

Tesofensine

Tesofensine was originally being designed as an Alzheimer's medication, and then they realized that many participants were losing weight! When looking at the low side effect profile compared to staying overweight; its easy to see why this compound is becoming a more popular option. For us, it really shines as our back-up option when someone is not medically qualified for Tirzepatide. Tesofensine users often report experiencing a significant reduction in appetite and an increase in weight loss, which could be attributed to Tesofensine's mechanism of action. It affects many components of brain chemistry: dopamine, serotonin, and norepinephrine. The combination leads to reduced physical hunger, less mental craving and even an increased metabolic rate.(73)

Another aspect of Tesofensine that has captured the interest of many is its potential to support metabolic health. By potentially improving insulin sensitivity and glucose metabolism, Tesofensine might contribute to better overall metabolic function, which could be particularly beneficial for individuals with type 2 diabetes or those at risk for developing the condition.(74)

Phentermine

Phentermine is a medication that can be used to help with weight loss. It is a stimulant that works by suppressing appetite and increasing metabolism. It's certainly not our go-to option, as the GLP1s medications are safer and more effective. But the way we utilize this medication is entirely unique. We recommend it be used for 3 days in a row max per week. While doing this, we work our patients into longer fasting windows as per the FLOA protocol; about 48 hours per week. If you desire the extra help but cannot get your hands on the GLP1-s, then this may be your next best option.

Most of the negative effects of Phentermine are associated with the daily use of it. That's what is so genius about our approach. We only use it as an aid to get into the FLOA and nothing more. That way, we avoid building a tolerance as well. Phentermine can help to maintain sufficient energy levels and suppress appetite during long fasting, which can be otherwise challenging. I can also improve mental clarity and focus that is also very helpful.

Contrave

Contrave is a prescription medication used to aid weight loss in adults who are overweight or obese. It is a combination of two active ingredients: naltrexone and bupropion. Naltrexone is primarily used to help patients who are dealing with withdrawal symptoms from alcohol and paid medications. In the context of weight loss, it's believed to affect the pathways in the brain that regulate appetite and food cravings. Bupropion is an antidepressant that's used to treat depression and prevent seasonal affective disorder. It can also help with quitting smoking. For weight loss, bupropion works by increasing certain types of brain activity, leading to increased levels of neurotransmitters (like dopamine) in the brain. This can help reduce appetite and increase energy expenditure

When combined, naltrexone and bupropion have a synergistic effect on weight loss, meaning their combined weight loss effect is greater than the sum of their individual effects. The exact mechanism of how these two drugs work together to enhance weight loss isn't fully understood, but their combination appears to impact areas of the brain involved in the regulation of appetite and energy expenditure.

It's all about getting into the rhythm of the long fasting. That is the ancestral wisdom part of things. And these medications are examples of science aiding us. Are they potentially harmful? Yes. But staying overweight is even more harmful, so we need to do whatever it takes. We will soon discuss just how we can wean

111

patients off these medications. But first, let's discuss some other powerful aids.

Artificial Induced Metabolic Flexibility

There are compounds that are generally much safer than medications and still much more powerful than supplements. Peptides are naturally occurring biological molecules composed of short chains of amino acids; the basic building blocks of our body. These molecules play a crucial role in numerous physiological processes, from hormone regulation and cellular repair to immune system function and tissue growth. Peptides are found throughout the human body, and their effects are as diverse as the cells and tissues they inhabit. Technically speaking, you can say the amino acids are no different from what you would find in any protein we eat or even collagen peptide supplements. Unfortunately, these products do not yield the same results. Wouldn't that be great! What makes peptide therapy yield these powerful results is the way they are three-dimensionally structured together. It's this specific structure that communicates a given action to another part of the body! There are over 7000 unique peptides identified to exist in the human body. Each plays a specific role in the overall function of your body, and together they are part of how the body attempts to maintain health and balance. Peptides are literal cellular languages. It's this reason why the side effect profile is almost nonexistent for most peptides. Pharmaceutical agents are all foreign to the body. One of the pioneers of peptide medicine: Dr. William Seeds, explains that this is why medications are so damaging and peptides are not. If doctors had all the peptides to choose from, they likely would never need a pharmaceutical agent again. But that's speculation on my part.

112

There are peptides that aid in the bodies' ability to mobilize body fat. The inability for the body to mobilize the fat fast enough is why many experience symptoms of low blood sugar when they start their fasting journeys. Earlier, we spoke about metabolic flexibility, which refers to the ability of your metabolism to burn both dietary fat and access the fat stores in your body effectively. The latter really means meeting the energy demands of your body. Maintaining weight does involve a lot of back and forth between fat burning and storage. But before the fat can be burned, it needs to be accessed or "mobilized." A high amount of metabolic flexibility means that in extreme situations, your body can still meet the energy demands by mobilizing enough fat fast enough to function optimally. What is more extreme of an energy demanding situation than not eating anything for 48 hours? Well, you can start adding some real workouts in the fasting window, but that's for when you become very metabolically fit. For the reader now, fasting alone is already intense enough

Notice my choice of words earlier.... "Mobilize enough fat fast enough to function effectively." It is in my opinion that the overwhelming majority of people are metabolically inflexible. Yet, despite this, they would all survive long periods of fasting. I can throw most of you on an island for 2–3 weeks and give you water and electrolytes, and you would all survive. But there is more that we need than to merely survive. We have work and life and manage many other responsibilities, so we require something that we can plug into life that doesn't overwhelm it so that we can actually accomplish it. When it comes to the symptoms of fasting: I have seen everything from extreme hunger, very low levels of energy, brain fog, and emotional swings.

Most people who start prolonged fasting will experience both hunger and exhaustion to a certain degree. It comes in waves and

113

FAST, FEAST, & FLOURISH

is unique to each individual. It really hasn't been researched enough to fully understand the mechanisms that explain such variance of response, but years of personal experience with myself and patients has given me a lot of insight and wisdom to the phenomenon. The energy crashing stems from your body's inability to maintain stable levels of blood glucose, and also from its inability to produce ketone bodies fast enough. Ketone bodies are the alternative source of fuel for your brain besides glucose. And they only get produced from a dietary intake free of carbs or fasting for long enough periods. This is why these peptides are so helpful. Remember, certain ones can aid in the mobilization of fat. So I like to think of them as "artificially induced metabolic flexibility."

The more prolonged fasting a person does, the more metabolically flexible they become. What matters here is this: the more prolonged fasting you do, the easier it will become to do more. But how do we get through the initial hump? How hard is the initial hump? It can be very challenging for the more unhealthy. But as you actually build more metabolic flexibility through fasting, it begins to get easier and easier. This is part of what sets you up for a future prolonged fasting. So let's live by one of my favorite quotes from Mr. Ben Greenfield and enjoy "better living through science."

AOD-9604

AOD9604 stands for "Anti-Obesity Medication." It is FDA-approved for weight loss. AOD is actually a fragment of the Human Growth Hormone(GH). Specifically, the part of it that aids in Fat Loss. This is our go-to peptide to complement Tirzepatide. AOD-9604 helps with metabolic flexibility by promoting fat breakdown and reducing fat storage. This could potentially lead to an increased ability for the body to utilize fats as an energy source, which is an important aspect of metabolic flexibility.(1)

CJC-1295/Ipamorelin

This is two different peptides combined that are commonly compounded together. These peptides are referred to as GH secretagogues. They stimulate the pituitary gland to release its stores of growth hormone. The combination of both produces a more potent release of As we age and begin to have lower levels of GH, it's not our production that is the issue, it's the signal to release it from the pituitary that decreases. There are many peptides in this category, but none are as safe and effective as the combination of these two peptides. In addition to its fat mobilization side, you also get all the other amazing benefits of increased growth hormone release, such as:

1. Improved muscle mass
2. Enhanced sleep
3. Better healing and recovery
4. Even strengthened immune function

We still prefer AOD over CJC/Ipamorelin as the primary focus is fast loss and AOD is better for that. But many of our patients enjoyed transitioning into CJC/Ipamorelin cycles when they hit their fast loss goals and looked to transition into a more physique optimization goal.

Concerns over GLP-1 Medications Long Term

We live in a very sick care system that unfortunately profits very heavily from us staying this way. There is much less money in preventive care for the pharmaceutical industry. With that being said, there is a time and place for everything. I do 100% acknowledge that there are situations for people where being on medication for the rest of their life may indeed be the best-case scenario for them. And I 100% respect those decisions. But I do believe that most people simply do not understand that there is a scenario where they maybe do not need to be on medication anymore. And they also don't know what it would take to create that scenario for themselves, aka address the underlying issues so that they would no longer require medicating. Doctors unfortunately won't get paid to educate on proper lifestyle interventions. They barely get paid as it is, which is why primary care physicians nowadays have to see such a high volume of patients to make ends meet. It's not the fault of the doctors, as they can only do so much in the small amount of time they get with you. They are also victims of a broken system

I've been on a mission to educate people on what it would look like for themselves to possibly create the changes needed to decrease the number of medications they have to take and help empower them to do so.

When it comes to GLP-1 medications, I find a great deal of confusion regarding their safety. There are earlier GLP-1 medications that have been out for decades. The first GLP-1 receptor agonist was eventide, which was approved by the US Food and Drug Administration (FDA) in April 2005 for the treatment of type 2 diabetes. This version and many others around its time required daily injections. The first GLP-1 to require only a weekly injection was Ozempic, which was barely FDA approved in 2017. There is a big assumption that seems to be going around that the safety studies for these earlier short-acting versions apply to these longer acting, more powerful ones. This is simply not the case. These drugs are required to go through their own long term safety studies. They can likely use the date from earlier versions to help accelerate the process, but new research must be done. It's a different compound which creates different effects. Effects we don't fully understand yet. There are GLP-1 receptors in many other organs in the body. We have no clue what the long-term ramifications of stimulating those receptors will be. Even if we had the long-term safety studies on semaglutide itself, which we don't, we have experienced many times in the past when medications were pulled off the market after being fully FDA approved and having long term safety studies. Here are a few examples:

1. Seldane (terfenadine): Seldane was an antihistamine medication that was approved by the FDA in 1985. It was later pulled off the market in 1997 due to reports of serious heart rhythm abnormalities (75).
2. Vioxx (rofecoxib): Vioxx was a non-steroidal anti-inflammatory drug (NSAID) that was approved by the FDA in 1999. It was later pulled off the market in 2004 due to an increased risk of heart attacks and strokes (76)
3. Baycol (cerivastatin): Baycol was a cholesterol-lowering medication that was approved by the FDA in 1997. It was later pulled off the market in 2001 due to reports of serious muscle damage and kidney failure (77)
4. Propulsid (cisapride): Propulsid was a medication used to treat gastrointestinal disorders that was approved by the FDA in 1993. It was later pulled off the market in 2000 due to reports of serious heart rhythm abnormalities
5. Redux (dexfenfluramine): Redux was a weight loss medication that was approved by the FDA in 1996. It was later pulled off the market in 1997 due to reports of serious heart and lung problems.(78).
6. Duract (bromfenac): Duract was a pain medication that was approved by the FDA in 1997. It was later pulled off the market in 1998 due to reports of serious liver damage (79).
7. Posicor (mibefradil): Posicor was a medication used to treat high blood pressure that was approved by the FDA in 1997.

It was later pulled off the market in 1998 due to reports of serious heart rhythm abnormalities. (80).

8. Rezulin (troglitazone): Rezulin was a medication used to treat type 2 diabetes that was approved by the FDA in 1997. It was later pulled off the market in 2000 due to reports of serious liver damage.(80).

9. Meridia (sibutramine): Meridia was a weight loss medication that was approved by the FDA in 1997. It was later pulled off the market in 2010 due to an increased risk of heart attacks and strokes.(80).

10. Bextra (valdecoxib): Bextra was an NSAID that was approved by the FDA in 2001. It was later pulled off the market in 2005 due to an increased risk of heart attacks and strokes.(80)

I want to be clear that the FDA is usually correct about approving a medication and letting us know that it's safe. But millions of people pay the price with their health and their life when they are mistaken. This is why drugs should be respected and only used when truly indicated. Furthermore, we should be encouraging people to take responsibility for their health. Questions like "what would it take to address the underlying issues of which this medication is simply masking for me at this time?" I'm very passionate about helping to educate people about this very thing. So here are my concerns over long-term use of the popular GLP-1 Medications. Many of these things can be found directly on the website of these medications themselves.

https://www.mounjaro.com/hcp

Pancreatitis

Pancreatitis is not a condition to be taken lightly. This little organ is responsible for producing the digestive enzymes our body needs to break down the food that we consume to be able to absorb the nutrients. This condition is inflammation of the pancreas, meaning it's damaged and possibly leaking the powerful digestive juices into areas we certainly do not want them. When looking at various studies to get an idea of how fatal acute pancreatitis can be, you will see ranges from 2% to 20% or even higher mortality rates. (81) There are obviously tons of variables, the biggest being how severe the pancreatitis is. But 2% is not negligible if you ask me.

From the literature, It is difficult to ascertain the exact % of people who started these GLP-1 medications and developed pancreatitis from it. From what I have researched, it may be pretty close to the placebo. This is great news for those looking to use it. But it can elevate your pancreatic enzymes. Clinically, we know elevated enzymes in labs are a potential indication of the early development of acute pancreatitis. I have personally seen this in our patients throughout the years. When this happens, we stop the medication to play it safe. You can find this on the website of Norvo Nordisk itself; the makers of Semaglutide:

Acute Pancreatitis: Acute pancreatitis, including fatal and non-fatal hemorrhagic or necrotizing pancreatitis, has been observed in patients treated with GLP-1 receptor agonists, including semaglutide. Acute pancreatitis was observed in patients treated with Wegovy® in clinical trials. Observe patients carefully for signs and symptoms of acute pancreatitis (including persistent severe abdominal pain, sometimes radiating to the back, and which may or may not be accompanied by vomiting). If acute pancreatitis is suspected, discontinue Wegovy® promptly, and if acute pancreatitis is confirmed, do not restart

Thyroid Cancers

Thyroid C-cell tumors, also known as medullary thyroid cancer (MTC), are a rare type of thyroid cancer that forms in certain cells of the thyroid gland. MTC accounts for 1-2% of thyroid cancers in the United States and is different from other types of thyroid cancers because it originates from the cells which produce the hormone calcitonin. (82) MTC's are usually more aggressive than other common types of thyroid cancer, and are easier to treat and control if found before it spreads to lymph nodes in the neck or other parts of the body. Thyroid function tests such as TSH are often normal, even when MTC's are present. The primary treatment for MTC's is surgery to remove the thyroid gland and surrounding lymph nodes. Elevated levels of calcitonin in the blood can indicate MTC at a very early stage. On their website and on the box, you will find this:

In rodents, semaglutide causes dose-dependent and treatment-duration-dependent thyroid C-cell tumors at clinically relevant exposures. It is unknown whether Wegovy® causes thyroid C-cell tumors, including medullary thyroid carcinoma (MTC), in humans as human relevance of semaglutide-induced rodent thyroid C-cell tumors has not been determined

In my opinion, the risk is very low here, and we will likely find out later that there is no potential for thyroid cancer in humans. But until then, we don't know. You would think that would be a requirement to know before a medication is FDA approved?? I suppose you can make the argument that the lives saved are worth the risk?

120

Regaining weight after stopping the medication.

We already mentioned in the very start of this book that about 70% of patients who lose weight from Semaglutide will regain the weight back within a single year after stopping. I saw that one coming a mile away when I first learned about this medication years ago. Look, this is the case for most weight loss medications. You now understand why that is. Your body's weight set point is a powerfully driven mechanism that is ultimately governed by Insulin. We get so many calls from people every single day searching for help with getting off the medication. The majority of them had no clue about the high likelihood of weight regain after stopping the medication. They were never told this. They were looking for a little "jump start." They either got it online at some research company, or they got it from a med spa and never even spoke to an actual doctor or had a very brief conversation with no guidance whatsoever!

We are very upfront with our patients about what the literature shows regarding the efficacy of this drug alone. That is why we do not provide this medication without co-current coaching from us. It goes against our integrity otherwise to simply provide the medication, especially given the clear statistics of rebound weight gain. Every day, we turn down patients who only want the medication and who do not share the same goal of short-term use only. They don't have to believe us at the start; they only need to trust us enough to give our program a go.

These medications are expensive

If you're opting for the pharmaceutical medications, you are looking to pay $1,000 – $1,500 per month. It's all fine and dandy when your insurance company is paying for it, but what happens if you lose your insurance or if your insurance stops covering the medication? Most people could not afford this ongoing bill for life, let alone for even a year. If you are working with a compounding pharmacy, receiving a product that has the same active ingredients Semaglutide or Tirzepatide, then you will likely be paying about $400 to $750 per month. I'm not saying that is cheap, either. But we're not advocating for using it longer than 3–9 months anyhow.

Why I am still a fan, but how do we use them

You may be wondering why I'm still a fan of GLP-1 use, given all of my concerns. Simply stated, I'm more concerned with the risks of staying overweight. Not just being overweight enough to be classified as obese, which is a designation of reaching a BMI of 35 or more. But even being mildly overweight has negative implications on your health. Health complications related to being overweight can start to manifest at different Body Mass Index (BMI) levels for different individuals. We discussed all that as well as why it gets harder and harder to break the cycle the more weight you gain earlier.

The initial barriers to fighting obesity are very challenging. Whether we are looking to start the FLOA protocol, or simply improve our eating patterns. Insulin resistance, chronic inflammation and a plethora of addictive foods all around us make it impossible for many to fight through the food chatter. These GLP-1s essentially reprogram our relationship with food, and they are powerful at doing so. With the food noise decreased and the powerful FLOA protocol in front of them; the results are now within reach.

What we are accomplishing with the FLOA protocol is absolutely wild. Despite what the literature suggests regarding the difficulty of maintaining weight after utilizing the medications; our happy patients have a different story to tell. The most significant part of our program is the ability for our patients to keep the weight off

AFTER stopping the medications. You now understand all the mechanics of how that's possible, and the following chapter will discuss implementation

Scan the QR Code to view Testimonials:

Let's Work With What I Got or What I Can Afford

I have helped thousands of people lose weight and maintain it without the use of medications or the peptides. We have a global wide program where I coach patients in a group setting every week on implementation of the FLOA protocol. It's a wonderful community of people across the world who are implementing the FLOA protocol with or without medications or peptides. At the end of the day, it's the FLOA protocol that is the magic; everything else is just an aid. Ultimately, It comes down to three things: how much help you want/need, what can you afford, and what do you have access to? Some people live in areas where they cannot access the GLP-1 medications or peptides. We have powerful supplement options that are available to ship globally, and these options can totally work as well. The proper mindset will always come into play for either program but matters even more when not using the stronger support. We will dive into the proper mindset later on. But first, let's review those the best supplements I have found over the past to help anyone implement the FLOA protocol.

Super concentrated Yerba maté tea or Unimate

Yerba maté tea comes from the leaves of the Ilex Paraguariensis plant, also known as the holly plant, which is native to and exclusively found in southern Brazil, northern Argentina, Paraguay, and Uruguay. (83) The dried leaves, twigs, and stems of this plant are used to prepare the beverage, which is widely consumed in South America. Yerba maté tea has been shown to have appetite-suppressing effects and potential benefits for weight loss and weight management. In one study, the consumption of Yerba maté promoted weight loss, attenuated the detrimental effects of a high-fat diet on adiposity and insulin sensitivity, and decreased blood levels of inflammatory biomarkers. (84) Another study found that Yerba maté treatment affected food intake, resulting in higher energy expenditure and lower body weight gain. (85) Additionally, a botanical composition composed of Morus alba, Yerba maté, and Magnolia officinalis demonstrated marked acute hypophagia (reduced food intake).(86) In this study on humans, they found that consumption of Yerba maté was associated with reductions in serum cholesterol, serum triglycerides, and blood glucose concentrations. (87)

There are a few problems with straight Yerba maté tea. First, it tastes pretty bitter and can be an acquired taste. Two, you have to drink a lot of it to get the desired effects. This is where Unimate Tea really shines. It is a concentrated Yerba maté tea product that mixes easily with cold or hot water, and it tastes great. It can be consumed at any time of day which makes it a flexible option for individuals following different fasting schedules. Whether you require a morning pick-me-up, a pre-workout boost, or an afternoon refresher, Unimate tea is quick and convenient

By curbing hunger, it enables you to stick to your fasting schedule without constantly battling cravings. Moreover, Unimate Tea is a mood enhancer, which can be particularly helpful during fasting periods when irritability or mood swings may arise due to hunger. This means that not only will you feel less hungry, but you'll also be in a better mood throughout your fasting journey. Another advantage of Unimate tea is its ability to heighten mental clarity. Staying focused and productive during fasting periods can be challenging, but with Unimate tea, you'll find it easier to concentrate on your tasks and maintain your productivity levels.

Yes, this product is expensive if you are comparing it to plain old Yerba maté tea. But having to brew a ton of it, sip it all day to get enough effect and dealing with the bitter taste is why regular Yerba maté tea is very impractical and why I recommend this product to aid your fasting journey. You can take one every day and a 2nd if needed on your longer fasting days.

If you want to purchase this product scan the QR Code below:

Fiber supplementation or delicious tasting feel great

Fiber has been known for a very long time to support digestive health, and soluble fibers, in particular, help maintain healthy cholesterol and blood sugar levels. It also has a tendency to create fullness within the digestive tract due to Its quality of expanding in water. All of these factors will support weight loss efforts. It stands out from regular fiber supplements due to its unique formulation and additional benefits. Here are some specific aspects that make it superior to regular fiber supplements:

1. Patented fiber matrix: Unicity Balance contains a patented fiber matrix that includes a blend of soluble and insoluble fibers, bioactive plant compounds, polysaccharides, and micronutrients. This unique combination offers a more comprehensive approach to fiber supplementation

126

compared to regular fiber supplements, which typically only provide one or two types of fiber.

2. Appetite control: The soluble fibers in Unicity Balance help increase feelings of fullness and satisfaction, making it easier to stick to a diet and avoid overeating. Regular fiber supplements may not have the same appetite-curbing effects.

3. Blood sugar management: The fiber matrix in Unicity Balance helps slow down the absorption of carbohydrates, which can help maintain healthy blood sugar levels and prevent energy crashes. Regular fiber supplements may not have the same impact on carbohydrate absorption and blood sugar regulation.

4. Cholesterol reduction: Unicity Balance contains a blend of plant extracts and phytosterols called Bios Cardio Matrix, which helps reduce the absorption of cholesterol in the body. Regular fiber supplements may not provide the same cholesterol-lowering benefits.

5. Vitamins and minerals: Unicity Balance includes a unique blend of vitamins and minerals called Bios Vitamin Complex, which contributes to overall health and well-being. Regular fiber supplements typically do not contain additional vitamins and minerals.

6. Scientific research: Unicity Balance's effectiveness is backed by scientific research, including a study conducted by the Cleveland Clinic, which showed that the fiber portion of Unicity Balance is effective in reducing the risk for cardiovascular disease. Regular fiber supplements may not have the same level of scientific support

In the United States, dietary fiber intake is generally lower than the recommended levels. According to a study analyzing data from the National Health and Nutrition Examination Survey (NHANES)

2009-2010, only a small percentage of the population met the adequate intake (AI) for fiber. Among adults who met the AI for fiber, major food sources included grain products, vegetables, legumes, and fruits. (88) As you start the FLOA protocol, you are dramatically decreasing your opportunity to eat fiber rich food. Which is why it's a good idea to supplement your fiber intake. Regular fiber supplements are still effective. But as you can above, the balance is better. But the best part is that it tastes freaking great. The normal instruction to use Balance is 15 minutes before you eat your two main meals on eating days. This is especially a must if you are not taking any GLP-1 medications, which suppress your appetite 7 days per week.

You can also take the Balance on your fasting days, during times of extreme hunger, in an effort to help you get through it.

Bitter extracts and appetite suppression aka Calocurb

Research on bitter compounds and appetite suppression has shown that these compounds can affect calorie intake and the release of appetite-regulating hormones. For example, a study demonstrated that release of a bitter compound, quinine, significantly affected calorie intake and cholecystokinin (CCK) release after a standardized meal.(1) CCK is a powerful appetite producing hormone and quinine was shown to lower it. Another study found that Amarasate™, a bitter hops-based appetite suppressant, reduced hunger during a 24-hour water-only fast. (89) The appetite-suppressing effects of bitter compounds are likely associated with gut peptides such as glucagon-like peptide-1 (GLP-1), cholecystokinin (CCK), and peptide tyrosine (PYY) (89)

Calocurb is a natural weight loss supplement that contains these bitter extracts. Taking it makes fasting easier by helping to manage cravings, hunger, and portion control. I haven't found any other product with these extracts in them. You can find some bitter orange containing products, but there is some evidence that it may increase blood pressure.(90) Flexible dosing options allow Calocurb to be tailored to your individual fasting schedule. For example, taking one Calocurb capsule at 9 am can help you complete your fast without hunger pains until noon. You can continue to take Calocurb throughout the day (at least 4 hours apart, with a maximum of 4 capsules per day) to control your portion sizes during your eating window and manage cravings when your eating window finishes. While fasting and using Calocurb, it's essential to keep your fluid intake high. Staying hydrated is crucial for overall well-being and can help alleviate some of the side effects of fasting, such as headaches or dizziness

For a link to purchase this product scan the QR Code below:

Nicotine without the bad parts

I know what you may be thinking, but hear me out. Nicotine can be a potential aid if used properly. Several human studies have investigated the effects of nicotine on appetite suppression. One study found that nicotine suppresses appetite and decreases food intake, leading to reduced body weight.(91) Another study demonstrated that nicotine could reduce appetite by affecting the activity of neurons in the brain that affect hunger.(92)

But I'm not recommending anyone take up smoking for weight loss. We clearly understand how dangerous tobacco use is. What I am pointing to is nicotine use without tobacco; Nicotine isolated. Nicotine in this form may be safe. There are studies on the safety of nicotine gum for non-smokers, although they are limited in number. One study investigated the effects of nicotine gum on psychomotor performance in non-smokers and found no significant drug effects in the non-smoker group.(93) Another study, the ENIGMA-Vis trial, aimed to investigate the effects of nicotine gum on vision in healthy non-smokers. The trial compared two doses of nicotine gum (2 mg and 4 mg) and a placebo gum in a randomized, double-blind, placebo-controlled trial.(93)

Nicotine has been shown to have nootropic effects, which means it can enhance cognitive function, including memory and learning. Some studies have investigated the effects of nicotine on memory and learning in animal models, such as rats. (94) In these studies, low doses of nicotine were found to improve learning and memory in adult rats, providing support for further investigation into nicotine as a potential therapeutic agent for diseases affecting cognition, such as Alzheimer's disease. Dr. Andrew Huberman is a neuroscientist and professor at Stanford University who's well known for his contributions to the fields of brain development, brain function, and neural plasticity. He acknowledges that nicotine can be a cognitive enhancer and has neuroprotective properties but advises against vaping and smoking forms of it.

Nicotine is a highly addictive substance, and its use can lead to dependence. It is not recommended if you were ever a prior smoker. If it were to be considered, it should be used in the same manner we looked at Phentermine. A means of helping us get into longer fasting periods, so a max of 2–3 days per week for periods of 2 months or so max. Start off very slow to assess tolerance. The lower dose gums are 2 mg. I recommend that you start at ¼ to ⅓ of this dose. I tried 2 mg myself the first time and wasn't too happy when I was throwing up on a flight that I was hoping to be studying literature on. Start slow and work your way up.

Other natural appetite suppressants

I separate the options below because while they are worth mentioning; they pale in comparison to the options above. If you aren't able to get your hands on powerful GLP-1 medications for whatever reason, then you may need all the other support you can get. The base would consist of the above options and any amount of the following as well.

1. Garcinia Cambogia: This tropical fruit extract is believed to help with appetite suppression and weight loss by inhibiting the enzyme that converts carbohydrates into fat. Typically, dosed between 500-1500 mg per day, taken 30-60 minutes before meals.(95)
2. Glucomannan: This natural dietary fiber derived from the root of the konjac plant can help promote a feeling of fullness and reduce overall food intake. About 1 gram, taken 3 times per day with a glass of water, 15-30 minutes before meals. (96)
3. 5-HTP: 5-Hydroxytryptophan is a naturally occurring amino acid that is a precursor to serotonin, a neurotransmitter involved in regulating appetite. Some studies suggest that

5-HTP supplements may help with appetite suppression and weight loss. The suggested dosage for 5-HTP is typically between 50-300 mg per day, taken in divided doses. (96)

4. Caffeine: Caffeine is a stimulant that can help increase metabolism and suppress appetite. It is commonly found in coffee, tea, and many weight loss supplements. A common recommendation is to consume 100-200 mg of caffeine per day, which is equivalent to 1–2 cups of coffee. (96)

5. CLA (Conjugated Linoleic Acid): CLA is a naturally occurring fatty acid found in meat and dairy products. Some studies suggest that CLA supplements may help with appetite suppression and weight loss. The recommended dosage for CLA supplements is typically between 3–6 grams per day, taken in divided doses with meals. (96)

6. Caralluma Fimbriata: This succulent plant has been traditionally used in India as an appetite suppressant and is now available in supplement form. The suggested dosage for Caralluma Fimbriata is typically 500-1000 mg per day, taken in divided doses. (97)

7. Fiber-rich foods: Foods high in fiber, such as whole grains, fruits, vegetables, and legumes, can help you feel fuller for longer periods, thus reducing hunger and aiding in fasting. (97)

8. Protein-rich foods: Consuming protein-rich foods like lean meats, fish, eggs, and dairy products can help increase satiety and reduce overall food intake. (97)

9. Healthy fats: Foods containing healthy fats, such as avocados, nuts, seeds, and olive oil, can help promote a feeling of fullness and support fasting efforts. (97)

10. Water: Drinking water before meals can help reduce hunger and overall food intake. (97)

11. Spices: Some spices, such as cayenne pepper and ginger, have been suggested to help suppress appetite and increase satiety. (97)

I don't recommend green tea extracts, as it's likely that it doesn't provide additional benefits that you wouldn't already be getting from the Unimate tea. There are obviously many options available when it comes to appetite suppressing supplements. You don't need to try them all. I recommend starting with the base of the more powerful ones I mentioned earlier and then experimenting with other options until you find the right stack that aids you in your FLOA fasting journey. As stated many times before, it will get easier over time, but utilize as much help as you desire to get you started. With all that being said, there is mental toughness to gain from doing it with less or no support. A lot of you will be challenging yourself even with the support, make no mistake, but if it starts off effortlessly, and you desire maximum mental toughness training, then try it with water only. The worse that will happen is you get back to needing support. Though most of you probably feel that life is already challenging enough as it is; I just wanted to mention that potential benefit if desired. Be sure to stay seated folks because the time is finally upon us. I'm proud to announce the FLOA protocol coming up next.

Part Four:
Welcome to the FLOA Protocol

Welcome to the culmination of my two decades of experience with shedding excess weight and achieving lasting results. I say with unwavering confidence that this is the final weight loss program you'll ever need. Throughout these years, I've not only guided countless clients and patients but have personally experimented with various methods.

Our collective struggles stemmed from misconceptions about obesity's mechanics and the daunting challenge of sustaining weight loss. My fundamental principle for success is to simplify, making it as straightforward as possible. As you embark on our program, I encourage you to reduce strenuous workouts and free yourself from the calorie-counting burden. There's no need to adhere to overly restrictive food lists. The easier we make the weight loss process, the less stressful and more sustainable it becomes. Remember, this isn't just another diet; it's a lifestyle shift—one that's remarkably achievable for our shared goals.

Prepare for an extraordinary journey. What I've crafted here is nothing short of the world's most aggressive and effective prolonged fasting protocol. I've introduced a structure where it was missing, a structure honed through personal trial and error. Reflecting on my journey, I often wonder if I would have embraced this approach with patients without first experiencing its transformative power on myself. While it's certainly possible, I believe my journey began in the early days of intermittent fasting, when it was a new frontier in the realm of health and wellness. This gave me a good head start and allowed me to take a deeper dive with patients back then. Ultimately, it all led to this: The FLOA protocol.

The core objective of the FLOA protocol is sustainable, genuine weight loss. For some, achieving long-term weight loss has remained an elusive dream. Others have never witnessed significant weight loss to begin with. FLOA delves deep into the underlying hormonal factors at the heart of obesity. We recognize the profound impact of genetics and how many of us have been dealt a challenging hand in this regard.

Fixing the Prior Metabolic Damage, aka the Weight Loss Plateau

A metabolic plateau, also known as a weight loss plateau, is a period during a weight loss journey when an individual's weight loss rate decreases or stops entirely despite continuing to follow the same plan that was working before. This phenomenon is common and eventually happens to most people who try to lose weight. Within the body, a plateau occurs when calorie expenditure equals intake over time, meaning the calories consumed equal the calories burned, and the calorie deficit no longer exists. Plateaus are a common occurrence in reaction to a calorie deficit over time. The body perceives a sustained calorie deficit over time as a threat to survival. It responds by closing the gap through a reduction in the basal metabolic rate (BMR) and non-exercise activity thermogenesis (NEAT). Essentially, this is a reduction in the number of calories we burn outside of exercise. It will also increase the drive to eat. Great survival mechanism; frustrating weight loss barrier for many. A plateau is a progressive process, and identifying one and course correcting is vital for long-term success. Pushing through a plateau by continuing on with deeper caloric restriction over time will only be met with stronger resistance from the body and a deeper plateau. (98)

I have worked with patients who have been in such wrecked metabolic situations, such as living off 800/900 calories per day. Pretty wild when you consider that a healthy TEE for a woman is somewhere around 1700-2400. It's wild how the body can survive off ½ the number of calories it would otherwise prefer. I like to call this "battery saving mode." The crazy thing is that the literature shows you would actually live longer in this state. (99) Battery saving mode is annoying to most of us. The laptop is not as fast, doesn't run as many applications at the same time, doesn't have as bright of a screen and goes to sleep much sooner than we appreciate. In humans, it actually isn't that much different. In this state, we have foggier thinking, lower energy, hair loss, constipation, aching body, intolerance to cold etc. Does that sound any fun to anyone?

Assessing if you are in one

We need to assess if you are in a current Weight Loss Plateau before starting any more weight loss. Some of these sound redundant, but you would be surprised how only one of them may resonate with people. It would be a great idea for everyone to start some sort of reset, but the excitement to get started for most pushes this idea to the curb. So let's look at 5 common ways to tell if you need to do this:

1. The obvious one is that you were losing weight and, with no change from your efforts, you are now losing less or none.
2. If you have been on a GLP1 medication for a month or more, then you are likely in some sort of compromised metabolic situation. Even if weight loss is still happening upon starting this program. Has it slowed down at all? The majority of people on these medications are enjoying the benefits of

daily appetite control, but are not aware of the effects of consistent caloric restriction.

3. You were losing weight in the past, and it stalled, and you have been stuck there for however long. Many times you answer "no" to #1 because the weight loss was so long ago. But if we looked at your calorie intake now, we would see how much less you are eating than what your TEE actually is supposed to be.

4. You have been in a caloric deficit for a long time. Maybe you tried to lose weight in the past but lost very little weight, and like #3 have been stuck there.

5. You are dealing with lower energy, brain fog, constipation, hair loss, ache bodies, intolerance to cold, and you recall that it seemed to have started sometime after starting your weight loss journey in the past.

6. If you are uncertain about being in one; it's always best to do a reset and err on the side of caution. Maybe you start counting calories after one week and realize you have been eating much more than you realized, and if so, then a reset may not be needed.

Figure out how many calories you have been averaging and compare it to where you should be at. This is a decent calculator, although I have always tended to see it about 1.2x higher than reality. It's still a decent gauge, though. You can find it at https://tdeecalculator.net/

How to fix it

1. You will need to count your calories during your reset. If you have no experience with how to do this, then find some videos on YouTube. I recommend using the app My Fitness Pal to help you with tracking.

2. Using your calculated average daily intake from the prior couple of weeks, slowly increase your calories, about 100-200 per week. Do this until you hit somewhere in the range of 80-90% of what the calculator said is your TEE.
3. Weekly weigh-ins are crucial here. You will likely stay at the same weight or even begin to drop weight as you increase your caloric intake.
4. Confirm success through two metrics
   a. Stable weight or weight decrease each week.
5. Improvement in symptoms. Pay attention to how you feel overall with the increase in calories. Be sure to document somewhere. You will likely begin to feel better regarding:
   a. Brain Fog
   b. Energy/tiredness
   c. Improvement in any of the symptoms discussed earlier.
6. The goal is to hit the ceiling! What does this look like?
   a. Constant weight gain
   b. Getting closer to the TEE calculators
7. Things to keep in mind.
   a. You can do stage 1 fasting, explained in the protocol, but do not do any more fasting beyond this amount. We have to focus on the reset first!
   a. The Keto diet is critical here. We want to minimize fat gain, and keto will help.
   b. Should you stop your GLP-1 medication during a reset? You will need to discuss with your prescribing physician. But I don't see any benefit of staying on it. In fact, it can make eating more difficult.
   c. Take a good mental note of what it looked like for you to be eating at your TEE. Since you won't be counting calories every single day, we need as much of a benchmark idea as possible. And now is the perfect

138

time to do so. Additionally, if you will be starting a GLP-1 or getting back on, then you really need to hit your TEE on a non-long fasting day to prevent another plateau,
    d. Resets can take 2–5 weeks, but the average is 3.

Due to the popularity of the GLP-1 medications, it's a very common occurrence for us to work with patients who have already lost 1/2 or more of their desired weight loss. They experience weight gain immediately when trying to wean off the medication, and saw one of our videos explaining how we have a successful format for helping people wean off. The reset is an integral part of the equation.

Understanding How We Should Approach Food

When I mentioned the importance of keeping it simple, I was mainly referring to the food part. Food has always been the bigger part of the diet vs. exercise equation. Because the FLOA protocol is so powerful, clinical observation has taught me, it allows for a lower level of discipline towards your diet while still yielding results. I must emphasize that it's not a ticket to eat whatever you want when you're not on your long fast. Now you understand that the exercise part as well as the quantity of calories doesn't matter as much as you had thought before. What matters most is optimizing your hormones if any lasting weight loss is desired. And by "optimizing," we really mean lowering your chronically elevated insulin levels. That's all it will take for the majority of you reading this. There are several other key things to address that will be necessary for some. Inflammation is one of the biggest after insulin control. Earlier you learned about how detrimental excess inflammation can be. Diet is hands down the biggest contributor to excess inflammation for most people.

So it sounds like "what" you eat may be of some pretty big importance to you.

Controlling insulin levels by doing Keto the smart way

The best way to thwart insulin in its tracks when you're not fasting is to take a ketogenic approach. We spoke in great detail earlier about how these diets failed in the long term but looked wonderful on the front end. So we are going to make out like a bandit with the perks while avoiding the downside. Sounds incredible, doesn't it? Really, all I mean is that we won't rely on the effects of keto in the long term to maintain the lower levels of insulin needed for easier weight maintenance. Instead, we will use it on the frontend only. It can also be an effective tool to use at times in the future. Many call this approach a cyclic keto diet.

Yes, there is such a thing as healthy keto vs. not. But if you take a keto approach towards the Paleo and/or Mediterranean diet, you are essentially doing that. We will talk more about these categories shortly. While you won't need to count your macros, it may help to estimate and visualize. 60-80% of your calories should come from fat. This diet is commonly mistaken for a high-protein diet, but it's not. Protein should have been 20-30% of your diet before, and it should remain the same. You are swapping carbs for healthy fats. To keep things simple, you will be doing this automatically when choosing fatty foods from the Paleo/Mediterranean categories. Approaching a keto diet is easier if you understand some things about the different types of fat that exist.

Fats can be broken down into three categories: saturated, monounsaturated and polyunsaturated. Structurally speaking, the difference lies in the presence of a double bond; Bond, James Bond.

140

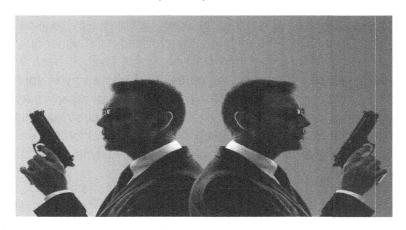

While all fat is the same in terms of the amount of energy it supplies per gram, the effects on your health are extremely diverse between the types. Entire books are written about this. We were taught that fat is bad, and that specifically saturated fats were the worst. Remember the American Heart Association, whose president had a heart attack at 52? Yea, these were the experts we have been listening too 😄 I hope you don't think I use this fact as the basis of my argument to discredit their advice. I just enjoy a good chuckle, and this joke never gets old. But back to the fats. The research is conflicting, with many experts advocating entirely different approaches. The approach I've landed on through decades of research and the last decade of working with patients and analyzing functional blood chemistry panels is a healthy mix of all three.

I recommend ⅓ of your fat intake comes from each category. Most experts agree the mono and polyunsaturated sources are good for you. But the controversy lies in the consumption of saturated fat. It is also important to mention that the delicious tasting fats tend to come from the saturated category. This is all your animal and dairy sources. Applying the principles of the damaging effects of

141

processed foods, we need to focus on higher quality sources of saturated fats. So if the budget allows for it, opt for higher quality sources of meat. Free-range chicken, grass finished beef, wild caught salmon. All organic, of course. My favorite way to source this is through a service like butcher box. Opting for organic sugar-free almond or coconut milk over cow's milk is a good substitute. Without complicating things, just estimate and shoot for ⅓ of each. Become familiar with sources of fat and what type of fat they compose of.

You will be able to re-introduce carbs back into your diet when you hit the deep fasting stages that will be better explained soon. Even if you want to do keto for longer, I don't recommend it unless you absolutely need to. For example, all else is implemented, and weight loss is not budging. The reason I want you to reintroduce carbs is simply because in the FLOA protocol you can have your cake and eat it too. Most people cannot stick to a keto diet long term. This is a crucial step here, so pay attention. This is why millions of people failed long term with the Atkins and ketogenic diets, and you won't. It was the diet only that was keeping insulin levels in check, so when they gave in and stopped eating a ketogenic diet, they quickly began to regain weight again. But the FLOA fasting is so powerful that most people will be able to have a life with carbs in it.

Give it about a month or two, and then you can start to re-introduce them back into your diet and enjoy this more sustainable lifestyle that you now get to live even while losing weight! Cycling through periods here and there where you lower your intake of carbs for a period of time is something that you do in the FLOA lifestyle. This is part of why maintaining weight will be so much easier for you.

Understanding fructose and the Insulin index

The current consensus among experts is that there is a link between fructose consumption and insulin resistance. Several human studies have investigated this relationship, and the evidence suggests that fructose intake may contribute to the development of liver insulin resistance by promoting fat production, impairing fat burning, inducing cellular stress, and triggering liver inflammation. (100) Increased fructose intake has also been associated with liver insulin resistance and fibrosis severity in nonalcoholic steatohepatitis which is essentially the damaging of liver tissue in later stages of fatty liver disease. (101)

High fructose corn syrup is the processed version of fructose. It became the staple of sweeteners used to replace sugar due to its cheaper costs and favorable effects of taste. Additionally, fructose has a lower glycemic index, so it was assumed it also had a negligible effect on insulin release. You should avoid high fructose corn syrup like the plague, as you are only going to find it in processed foods anyhow. More on the glycemic index and processed foods shortly. So in essence, as bad as sugar is for us, fructose on its own is worse because it will likely produce more insulin secretion than non fructose sugar would. This leads to faster development of insulin resistance. You already learned how nasty the back and forth between insulin resistance and chronically elevated insulin levels are

But fruit is the one that always enters the arena for discussion. You will find plenty of high-quality research advocating that fruit should be part of a weight loss program. You will also find a ton of literature supporting calorie restriction approaches as well, and the majority of you failed miserably with that. ☺

Fruit is not nearly as bad as high fructose corn syrup containing foods, no doubt, but when you are insulin resistant you are throwing gasoline on an insulin resistant fire. Most fruits, after consumption, will cause a larger release of insulin. We need to keep levels at bay to heal the insulin resistance. This means minimizing fruit intake at least during the weight loss phase and re-introducing back as you progress towards your goal. How can we understand which fruits are the worst culprits? Here comes the insulin index.

The insulin index is a scale that measures blood levels of insulin following a meal, allowing you to better understand your insulin response to certain foods. It is similar to the glycemic index (GI) and glycemic load (GL), but instead of relying on blood glucose levels, the insulin index is based on blood insulin levels. This index can be more useful than the glycemic index or glycemic load because certain foods, such as lean meats and proteins, can cause an insulin response despite having no carbs present. It's important to become familiar with this chart because insulin is just as damaging when it comes from lower glycemic foods. Some examples of foods that are high on the insulin index but lower on the glycemic index include:

1. Dairy products: Low-fat dairy products, such as yogurt and cottage cheese, can have a higher insulin index despite having a low glycemic index.
2. Lean meats: Foods like chicken and turkey can cause an insulin response, even though they do not contain carbs.
3. Fish: Certain types of fish, such as salmon and tuna, can also cause an insulin response despite having a low glycemic index.
4. Nuts: Although nuts are generally low on the glycemic index, some varieties, like peanuts, can have a higher insulin index.

144

Paleo/Mediterranean diet

I prefer the Mediterranean and/or Paleo approaches towards food choices.

The Paleo diet, which focuses on whole, unprocessed foods that humans might have consumed during the Paleolithic era, is known for its anti-inflammatory properties. By emphasizing the consumption of fruits, vegetables, lean meats, fish, eggs, nuts, and seeds, the Paleo diet eliminates many inflammatory food sources, such as grains, legumes, and dairy products. (102) This diet is rich in anti-inflammatory nutrients, such as omega-3 fatty acids and antioxidants, which can help combat inflammation and reduce the risk of chronic diseases associated with it, such as heart disease and metabolic syndrome. Fruits and vegetables, in particular, have been linked to lower levels of C-reactive protein (CRP), a marker of inflammation. (103)

Studies have indicated that the Paleo diet can lead to improved heart health, reduced inflammation, and weight loss. (104) By focusing on nutrient-dense, anti-inflammatory foods, the Paleo diet can support overall health and help manage inflammation-related issues. Moreover, the Paleo diet has been found to be the most anti-inflammatory diet among the 16 most popular diets in a peer-reviewed meta-analysis. By eliminating pro-inflammatory foods like refined carbs, dairy, and sugar, and incorporating anti-inflammatory foods such as avocados, berries, fish, green vegetables, leafy vegetables, nuts, seeds, olive oil, and tomatoes, the Paleo diet can help reduce inflammation and promote healthier aging. (104)

The Mediterranean diet is a primarily plant-based eating plan that emphasizes whole grains, olive oil, fruits, vegetables, beans, legumes, nuts, herbs, and spices. It includes animal proteins in smaller quantities, with fish and seafood being the preferred sources. This diet is known for its anti-inflammatory properties, which can help combat inflammation and ward off chronic diseases associated with it, such as heart disease, metabolic syndrome, and diabetes. The diet's focus on nutrient-dense, minimally processed, and locally grown foods makes it a sustainable and healthy option for long-term adherence. (105)

The effects of processed foods

These categories are not an exhaustive list by any means. But these categories help to give some initial structure to the overwhelming amount of information regarding what to eat to lose weight. What do they have in common? The fundamental key is to eat less processed foods, as these foods really screw you up in so many ways, such as:

1. High in calories, sugar, salt, and unhealthy fats: Processed foods often contain excessive amounts of these ingredients, which can lead to weight gain when consumed in excess. (106).
2. Low in essential nutrients: Processed foods tend to lack important vitamins and minerals, which can affect your ability to exercise and burn calories. A nutrient-poor diet may also prevent you from feeling full after eating, leading to overeating and weight gain. (106)
3. Highly addictive: Processed foods are designed to be addictive, increasing your appetite and making it difficult to stop eating them.(106)
4. Increased calorie consumption: Studies have shown that consuming ultra-processed foods can cause people to eat more calories and gain weight. In one study, participants ate about 500 more calories per day on an ultra-processed diet

and gained an average of 2 pounds over a two-week period. Calories seem to matter when in states of excess inflammation. (107)

5. Lack of satiety: Processed foods are typically stripped of nutrients and fiber, which can leave you feeling unsatisfied and more likely to overeat.(106).

Big business profits when you buy more processed food, and addicted customers drive the best business. We are blasted with marketing efforts. We are blasted with addictive chemicals. Furthermore, we were taught by the "experts" that this stuff was safe. Large food companies have funded research to promote their products or downplay the negative effects of certain ingredients. This can lead to biased research findings and potentially misleading information about the health benefits of certain foods.

For example, In the 1960s, the sugar industry funded research that downplayed the risks of sugar and highlighted the hazards of fat, according to newly published articles in JAMA Internal Medicine.(108) The sugar industry paid scientists to play down the link between sugar and heart disease and promote saturated fat as the culprit instead. (109) The sugar-funded project in question was a literature review, examining a variety of studies and experiments. It suggested there were major problems with all the studies that implicated sugar, and concluded that cutting fat out of American diets was the best way to address coronary heart disease.(108) The studies used in the review were handpicked by the sugar group, and the article, which was published in the prestigious New England Journal of Medicine, minimized the link between sugar and heart health and cast aspersions on the role of saturated fat. (110) The sugar industry trade group initiated and paid for the studies, examined drafts, and laid out a clear objective to protect sugar's reputation in the public eye.The sugar industry paid two

Harvard professors to point the finger elsewhere, and they cherry-picked the data and minimized the problems with sugar and maximized the problems with saturated fat. (109)

Similarly, Coca-Cola has funded research that focused on physical activity, thereby downplaying the role of sugar-sweetened beverages in obesity. (111) The American Society for Nutrition has accepted funding from companies like PepsiCo, Nestlé, Coca-Cola, and McDonald's to produce research that falls in favor of big food companies. These companies have been found to influence the research agenda by focusing on certain research topics, often related to single nutrients that can be manipulated by food companies.(111)

Trans fats

Trans fat is short for "partially hydrogenated fats." Trans fats can be classified into two categories: natural and artificial trans fats. Natural trans fats are found in small amounts in some animal products, such as meat and dairy, and are produced by bacteria in the stomachs of these animals. Artificial trans fats, on the other hand, are created through an industrial process called hydrogenation, which involves adding hydrogen to liquid vegetable oils to make them more solid. This process is used to increase the shelf life and improve the texture of processed foods. While trans fats are considered unsaturated regarding the 00 bond status; they should be avoided like the plague. They are awful and no one is auguring for their incorporation into your diet.

The literature is pretty clear on how detrimental it is to your health.(112) The primary sources of trans fats are: Fried foods, baked goods, margarine, shortening, fast foods, frozen meals, and processed snack foods. Are we seeing the trend here? The majority of culprits are the same processed crap we have been talking about.

Yet big fast food and restaurant chains won't stop serving it up. Big food and snack companies won't stop their efforts to sell you their highly addictive sh** That is chock-full of trans fats and a bunch of other crap.

Here are some of the effects of consuming this garbage regularly: (113)

1. Increased risk of heart disease: Trans fats raise LDL (bad) cholesterol levels and lower HDL (good) cholesterol levels, increasing the risk of heart attack or stroke.
2. Increased risk of type 2 diabetes: Trans fats are associated with a higher risk of developing type 2 diabetes, although the relationship is not completely clear.
3. Inflammation: Trans fats promote inflammation, which is implicated in heart disease, stroke, diabetes, and other chronic conditions.
4. Endothelial cell dysfunction: Consuming trans fats reduces the normal healthy responsiveness of endothelial cells, the cells that line all of our blood vessels.
5. Obesity and insulin resistance: In animal studies, eating trans fats has been shown to promote obesity and resistance to insulin, which is a precursor to diabetes.
6. Increased risk of certain cancers: Trans fats have been linked to an increased risk of breast, prostate, and colorectal cancers.
7. Adverse effects on brain and nervous system: Trans fats can be incorporated into brain cell membranes, altering the ability of neurons to communicate and potentially diminishing mental performance.

8. Increased risk of death: High trans fat intake increases the risk of death from any cause by 34%, coronary heart disease deaths by 28%, and coronary heart disease by 21%

Scary Sh** huh?! Does this mean we can never have any of this stuff again? The last thing I want to do is create extreme scenarios for people about food. I find it leads many people, down the path of "Ahh fu** it. You only live once." Trans fat is primarily found in processed foods, with a few outliers.

The 90/10 rule

I prefer a healthy relationship with food, and this means allowing for some of the horrible crap mentioned beforehand. Would it be wonderful for your health to eat the perfect diet? Absolutely! You would likely feel pretty spectacular doing so after your inflammation begins to decrease. Would it become easier and easier to adhere to the new lifestyle? For many, yes it would. The problem though is that crappy food is really addicting.(3) Ask most recovering addicts the same question, and most will tell you that it gets easier over time. But why do your friends who become Alcoholic Anonymous(AA) success stories rarely go out anymore and only seem to want to hang out with their new friends from AA? Because the success rate is much higher when you remove yourself from the vicinity of temptations. When your strategy for success involves complete abstinence, it requires you to continue doing so out of concern over an extreme binge-like reaction when accidentally breaking it. So, unless you plan to go live on a remote island with an abundance of clean food and not a Mickey Ds in sight; it's not so realistic that we can truthfully remove all the temptations of addictive food. I found, working with patients for so many years, that the more extreme they went in their diets, the greater likelihood they would let loose and resort back to a diet that was full of crap again. I lived this cycle myself and it's awful. Very emotionally challenging to say the least. But what I have noticed is that the less dramatic the change, the less dramatic the fall.

This is why I advocate for the 90/10 rule. We're looking to heal from the food addiction, while establishing that you can have a smaller amount of crappy food in your diet and still be successful. Let's keep it clean for 90% of the time. Then allow for 10% of whatever you want. Remember, we are also doing supercharged FLOA fasting alongside. This is why there is more leeway in the crappy food category.

I am fine with patients that want to go as close to 100% as clean as they can within say the first 3 months. There is some massive benefit to this for the more inflamed and/or insulin resistance types; they may even have too. In fact, when our patients are not responding, this is essentially the next step. But we continually strive to make it as easy as we can, and only make it more difficult if we need to. With a more extreme start like this, you should be in agreement with yourself that this is commitment, but for a defined period of time. Like 3 months, for example. And that you will allow yourself to slip into the 90/10 rule afterward if you desire to when you get there. If there is a self rewarded 75/25 week the first week afterward, that is also ok! The same concept here applies, attempting to make it less extreme. That way, if you do fall off the horse, it's easier for you to get back up!

If you suffer with an autoimmune disorder such as Hashimoto's disease, then the avoidance of inflammatory foods will be AS important as reducing insulin will be for successful weight loss; possibly more. You won't have as much wiggle room with your diet as others will. But I can tell you from personal experience that autoimmune patients do great when they get the diet part down. While a more strict adherence overall is needed, they still get the same benefit of a comparative decreased discipline that would be otherwise required due to what fasting does for inflammation produced from the autoimmune disease.

When it comes to food, we need to eat mostly unprocessed foods, follow a keto diet for the first 4–6 weeks and avoid high insulin index foods. When you are going to cheat, keep it under 10%. Outside your fasting windows, that's really it, and there's no need to overly complicate things here. Yes, we have wonderful science backed support to help us adhere to better food choices. But what I have also found to be very helpful as well is developing the proper mindset.

Develop the Right Mindset

The mind is a powerful tool. Just look up who David Goggins is and see for yourself a real life example of just how powerful the mind is. While this is an example of the extreme, it's also a look into our potential. A proper mindset can significantly contribute to weight loss success by influencing motivation, self-regulation, and self-efficacy. Developing a positive mindset can help you stay committed, make better choices, and overcome challenges during your weight loss journey. (114)

At Colorado Medical Solutions, we have had a specific patient come in for about the last 6 years – someone who instantly wins over the staff the moment she meets them. Let's call this patient "Mrs. D." Every day, when asked, "How are you doing today, Mrs. D?" she responds with something incredibly powerful:

"I woke up this morning, so I'm blessed."

Isn't it hard not to feel a bit jealous of this person? Don't we all kind of wish that we could wake up with that positive of a mindset? Just imagine how that could transform your life.

It's likely that this isn't your first attempt at losing weight. Through my years of experience, I've discovered that mindset plays a pivotal role in the success of any weight loss journey. No matter how meticulously planned your approach is, your ability to follow through ultimately determines your success. While our program is designed to minimize the need for a perfect mindset, it's still worth addressing

Have you ever set out to achieve something or break a bad habit and fall short? Often, this happens because people lack the structure needed to clarify their goals. These aspirations may float around in their minds, seemingly well-defined, but without clear documentation, they remain elusive

Start by finding a quiet, distraction-free space. Turn off your phone, close your eyes, and dedicate a few minutes to visualize your goals. Picture the ideal version of yourself. Release any inhibitions as you do this. Thoughts like "that's too ambitious" or "I don't need to be that fit" are protective mechanisms your brain deploys to shield you from potential failure. The prospect of striving for those goals and falling short can be intimidating, leading to these negative feelings and attitudes, especially for someone aiming for a six-pack while being significantly overweight or lean arms as a 100-pound overweight female. Overcoming these strong mechanisms may require effort, but remember, you control your mind, not the other way around. Once you've overcome these barriers, you'll see the true version of yourself that you desire. You should feel a surge of positivity at this point. If you haven't, it means you haven't fully conquered those mechanisms yet, so persist

Once you've reached this mental state, put your thoughts into writing. Describe in vivid detail how you envision yourself, to the extent that someone else could read your words and visualize the same image you've conjured

Even more crucial than crystal-clear goals are the "why's" behind them. Why do you want this transformation? Is it for improved health, to break free from the weight-induced slumps, to excel in a sport, to feel confident in your own skin, or perhaps to ensure you're there for your grandchildren as they grow? Write these reasons down. Then, delve deeper and keep asking yourself "why" until you reach the core motivation, the single "why" that drives it all. Its power cannot be overstated

Next, acquire a whiteboard and position it where you'll see it daily, perhaps near your bed or in your bathroom. Personally, I prefer it right next to my bed. I make a habit of reading these goals every morning and night, although I'm not perfect, and occasionally, I forget. Even during stressful periods when I might neglect them for a few days, I always return to this routine, mainly because the board is right there next to my bed – it's hard to overlook. This strategy applies effectively to all your goals, not just weight loss, but for now, let's concentrate on this aspect. Write your goal at the top, and beneath it, emphasize the "why" in larger letters. Remember, the "why" holds more significance than the goal itself

Affirmations are incredibly potent

Your brain is naturally programmed to filter out irrelevant information. However, affirmations serve as a tool to make anything important to your brain, even if it would typically be filtered out. Recall the last car you purchased, perhaps a Jeep Cherokee. After owning it, did you start noticing more Jeep Cherokees on the road? Did more people suddenly start driving them? Of course not, but before owning one, a Jeep held no more significance to you than any other car. Your Reticular Activating System, the part of your brain responsible for this filtering, is the reason behind this phenomenon. It's a valuable mechanism because, without it, you'd be overwhelmed by the over 14,000,000 bits of information bombarding you every moment. (115) Your brain focuses only on what truly matters. For instance, things related to family, work, or personal interests. Everything else gets filtered out. By consistently practicing these affirmations every morning and evening, you'll compel your brain to prioritize these goals, manifesting them into reality

I urge you to get a support system, someone to help keep you accountable. This can be your husband, wife, partner, boyfriend, girlfriend or just plain friend! Someone who you feel comfortable enough to share these things with. Let them see your goals. Ask them for help on keeping you accountable. Tell them what you are doing and what you are striving for, and ask for their support on this. This works great for people you spend a lot of time with, if that's possible. You'd be surprised how powerful this could be, even if all they did was re-read the goals that you wrote up yourself. This is because your attitude will constantly change. You will do your best to always keep a positive attitude, but you won't always be able to. Especially when you are not seeing results. That's when the support system really shines. A highly recommended book for you to have a deeper dive into the power of manifestation would be: Think and Grow Rich by Napoleon Hill.

*Takeaway to Never Forget: Find a support system and get someone to keep you accountable. Do this at all costs. Your likelihood of success will increase dramatically.

FLOA Fasting

Let's dive into the mechanics of FLOA fasting and what it actually looks like.

Stages of fasting

There are three stages of fasting, and your goal is to get to FLOA stage as comfortably or uncomfortably fast (speed wise) as you desire to do so. Are you a "rip the bandage off" kind of person? Or would you rather experience a lower degree of discomfort for a longer period of time? Ultimately, the choice is yours. It's important to understand that it's not that black and white. There are so many variables that will affect an individuals' difficulty of getting into the longer fasting stages. The biggest variables are:

1. Access to use medications and/or peptides.
2. Dealing with obesity genetics.
3. Current health status – how obese, insulin resistant and inflamed are you?
4. Mindset strength.

Many more variables exist as well. I mention these for you to not be discouraged, regardless of the outcome. If you do decide to rip the bandage off and experience massive bleeding, then simply put it back on. If you attempt a longer fast and cannot persist through the discomfort, then stop. Document how long that round was and beat it next time. If you prefer to peel it off, that is completely fine as well. The stages of FLOA fasting are:

1. Stage 1 – Time-restricted eating or intermittent(IF) – 16/8
   Choose a 6-9 hour eating window that ends at least three hours before bed and starts at least 2 hours after you wake.

2. Stage 2 – 24 hour fasting. In addition to the above, add two 24-hour fasts per week. Every 3 days or so. Even if you can't get to 24 on your first attempt, anything longer than stage one is progress. Once you can complete 2 24 hour fasts in the week with more ease, then you are ready for the big kahuna.
3. Stage 3 FLOA – 48 hours once per week. Same mentality as above. Document how long and beat it next week.

If you can start the FLOA stage and keep it up within the first few couples of weeks, then great! If you need a couple of months to work into that stage, that is also completely fine. All humans have this same metabolic system, and we are all built for this lifestyle of fasting. We are the genetic results of millions of years of evolution, where the humans who couldn't survive fasting like this died off and didn't end up contributing to our genetic make up today. Never get discouraged, as progress is progress

If you require additional help implementing the FLOA protocol, there are many levels of support available to you.

FLOA university; a series of online courses designed to better help you understand and implement the FLOA protocol. Better yet, if you would like to join the thousands of others in the FLOA community who participate in live group coaching, you can request information by scanning the QR Code below.

Planning Out the Schedule for FLOA Fasting

For simplicity, I recommend picking the same two days to fast on. Say Monday dinner until Wednesday dinner. While there's an argument to be made that it may be even better to alter the schedule, it's generally easier for people to stick to a schedule for the weekly long fast. Pick days when you can stay the busiest. Fasting is always so much easier when you can stay busy. It's important to stay as consistent as possible with your weekly weigh-ins. You should still record your weight, even if you forget and are off a day or two. Plan now, ahead of time, what part of the week you think your weekly long fast will be when you get to the FLOA stage. This is significant, so you can start your weekly weigh-ins now. You want your weigh-in date to be the day before or the AM you start your long fast. You should not be weighing yourself 12 hours or later into your fast!! When you fast, you will deplete your stored carbs (glycogen) and drop a lot of water weight, and it can make the weekly weigh-ins more difficult to interpret. For example, if you eat dinner Monday evening and start the fast afterward, your weekly weigh-in should be Monday or Tuesday AM.

Weekly weigh-ins are important to ensure you are on track with your goal. You should be losing about 1% of body weight per week. If you are, then there is no need to change anything. If you are losing more than 1/1.5% of body weight per week, you could technically decrease your FLOA fasting window by 12 hours or eat a bit more food on the non-fasting days. The fact that rapid weight loss has a strong correlation with rebound weight gain doesn't seem to apply with this approach. If you are losing over 1.5% per week, you are probably under eating on the other 5 days. The main reason this can happen is that the GLP-1 medications are so powerful, and you will be so motivated to keep the momentum going from the crazy fast results you will be seeing that you may desire not to force yourself to eat during the non-fasting days. By under-eating on non-fasting days, you do run the risk of your body triggering a metabolic weight loss plateau. Don't let this happen and ensure you eat enough!!! This is another reason the weekly self check-ins are great.

Supplements during your long fasting days

This does not need to be 0-calorie water fast. While that style of fasting will unlock some more of the health benefits and tap more into the cellular autophagy we spoke of earlier; it's something we can work on after we get to our goal weight. Eating less often and eating less food means a possibility of micro nutrient deficiencies.

So it is recommended to take your normal vitamins and supplements. Splash some sugar-free, dairy-free creamer in your coffee if you desire. The only brand I recommend is Nut Pods because it's sugar and dairy-free and low calorie. Oh yea, calorie-free drinks are ok, but only sweetened with monk fruit, stevia, or erythritol. Other sweeteners will likely spike insulin levels. One serving of sugar-free electrolytes sweetened with these sweeteners and ¼ tsp of salt needs to be added as well. You will drop a lot of water, so it's important to replace the lost electrolytes.

The supplement world is massive and overwhelming. It's easy to get lost in all the various things that are out there. What I put together is a basic list of 4 essential products that everyone should be taking for overall health:

1. High-quality fish oil – We simply do not get enough essential fatty acids in our diet. EPA (eicosapentaenoic acid) and DHA (docosahexaenoic acid) are essential omega-3 polyunsaturated fatty acids (PUFAs) that play crucial roles in maintaining overall health and supporting weight loss. They are vital for various physiological processes, including brain function, cardiovascular health, and inflammation regulation.(116) (117) **About 2–3 grams per day** is usually enough to get about 1 gram of the EPA and DHA that our bodies need each day.

2. Vitamin D – It is vital for calcium homeostasis and bone metabolism, which helps maintain strong bones and teeth. Vitamin D is also involved in immune system regulation and has anti-inflammatory properties. It also seems to help prevent diseases. Vitamin D deficiency has been linked to several health issues.(118) (119) (120) **Take 5,000IUs in the AM.**

160

3. Curcumin – A compound found in turmeric, has been shown to have potent anti-inflammatory properties. It can help regulate numerous factors and cytokines linked to inflammation, making it a potential therapeutic compound for various inflammatory diseases.(121) Some studies have demonstrated that curcumin can effectively improve symptoms of inflammatory bowel disease, psoriasis, atherosclerosis, and COVID-19.(121) A good dose is **525 mg curcumin 2x a day with 2.5 mg piperine (to enhance absorption) 2x/day**

4. Resveratrol, a polyphenolic compound found in foods like grapes, red wine, and berries, also exhibits anti-inflammatory effects. It has been associated with a reduced risk of cardiovascular diseases, cancer, liver diseases, obesity, diabetes, Alzheimer's disease, and Parkinson's disease.(122) Resveratrol's anti-inflammatory properties are attributed to its ability to modulate multiple cell signaling molecules.(123) A good dose is **250 mg 2x/day**

5. Magnesium – Magnesium has really grown in popularity in the more recent times. Like vitamin D, it plays an important role in multiple aspects of health. Potential cardiovascular benefits.(124) Magnesium has been associated with anti-inflammatory effects and improved vascular health. Weight loss support: In morbidly obese diabetic and non-diabetic patients, modest weight loss was associated with improved magnesium levels.(125) There are two forms of magnesium I recommend; glycinate and threonate. Threonate has a special added benefit of calming anxiety before bed. **About 2 grams of Threonate before bed and about 200 mg of glycinate in the morning.**

6. A daily multivitamin – Just some insurance over all micro nutrient needs.

Scan the QR Code for a direct link to purchase my recommended supplements:

Intermittent fasting on non-long fasting days

When you are FLOA fasting each week at 36+ it's not as important to get your 16-hour fast on the other five days. It will certainly help and is recommended as long as you get your total number of calories required as discussed earlier. If you are having a hard time eating on the GLP-1 medications during the other 5 days, then it's ok to expand the eating window on those days. When you are through your program and maintaining your weight via the FLOA lifestyle, then yes, daily intermittent fasting is significant since you won't be doing a long fast every week anymore.

Breaking the Fast

I recommend that you break a long fast with caution and mindfulness. When you fast, your digestive system goes into a deep repair mode. We know how amazing this is for our health, but we have to understand the ramifications of this and how to deal with it. During this time of deep repair, your body stops producing the enzymes necessary for proper digestion. It takes time for the system to "wake up" and be ready for proper normal digestion. The longer you fasted for, the longer the recovery period will need to be. For our typical 48 hours in the FLOA protocol, it will take about 24 hours to fully recover. In other words, you are eating in this "slightly altered state" for about 24 hours, after which you can resume normal eating.

During this 24-hour period, you need to start with the easiest to digest food and work your way into more difficult meals. The variables that affect digestion difficulty levels are:

1. Size of the meal
2. Amount of fat
3. Amount of processed crap
4. Presence of raw foods like veggies, nuts, and seeds.

All of these things require more effort from your digestive system. When it comes to your meals, think lean protein and steamed veggies. Soups are the best to break with your first meal, and bone broth is a favorite way to do this. Keep the portions small and eat periodically throughout the next 24 hours as you "wake up" your digestive system. After 12–16 hours into the post fast, you can start eating bigger, normal-sized meals. I still recommend you focus on easier to digest food, though. Listen to your body. The tell-tale sign that you ate too much or too fast or both is diarrhea, nausea, bloating, or indigestion like feelings. Every week is a new opportunity to learn more about your body and what it best responds to during the post fast stage. Over time, your body gets more adapted to coming out of longer fasts.

Food to break your fast with in somewhat order of complexity

1. Bone broth: It is easy to digest and contains essential minerals and vitamins
2. Soups: Soups containing protein and easily digestible carbs, such as lentils, tofu, or pasta, can gently break a fast. Avoid soups made with heavy cream or a large amount of high-fiber, raw vegetables
3. Cooked or steamed vegetables
4. Lean proteins
5. Fermented foods: Unsweetened yogurt or kefir can be gentle on the digestive system
6. Healthy fats: Foods like eggs or avocados can be great first foods to eat after a fast, but in small amounts.

When taking GLP-1 medications

Get enough calories on the non-long fasting days. I can't stress this enough! If you fast for 48 hours and then eat under your Total Energy Expenditure (TEE) for 5 days, you will hit a plateau and hit it fast! Gauge your intake compared to how you were eating before. You are to eat a minimum of that much for the five days. The patients that work with us, are submitting their weekly weigh-ins, so we can spot the plateaus before they develop. But if you are doing this on your own, then you really need to be cognizant of how you are eating these 5 days. The day after the 2 days is a build up day. So the other 4 days MUST BE AT YOUR TEE, or even a little higher is fine.

Calorie restriction over time creates a plateau

The bigger the calorie deficit, the faster you hit a plateau. People taking the GLP-1s and not doing the FLOA protocol experience this

164

all the time. They are severely under-eating each day due to the effects of these medications. But I'm teaching you now that you will likely need to eat more on those days than you will desire to if on these medications.

Should I count my calories? It's a lot of work and takes a decent amount of time. Everyone will benefit tremendously from the effort of going through this process, though. It gives you responsibility and appreciation for proper portion control. It's just that with this program, you won't have too. And that is actually part of what makes it so sustainable. If it doesn't sound stressful to you to do this for a few weeks, though, then you should totally do this. The weekly weigh in process tells us a lot. You can either change the fasting window length or the number of calories/amounts of food you are eating during the non-fasting days too. If you are losing too much weight as discussed earlier, then eat more during your non-long fasting days.

Alternate your FLOA fasting occasionally

The body is a constantly adapting machine looking for the most efficient way to go about doing things. It learns from prior experiences to accomplish efficiency. This is similar to the concept we discussed earlier, where the body prefers to maintain a state of balance or homeostasis. If you fasted for 48 hours every single week for the rest of your life, I do believe it would lose a good portion of effectiveness. One of our favorite benefits is the lowered discipline it affords you. To keep it going, it's a good idea to keep your body guessing and to switch things up preemptively. Most gym-goers know that you need to eventually switch up your routine for continual gains of muscle development, and fasting is likely no different.

I recommend switching up your fasting on average once per month, but it certainly can be more often. If you have a crazy schedule, let that schedule naturally switch things up for you. You can do things like:

1. A maximum of a 72-hour fasting period.
2. 2 36's in a week.
3. 3 24's in a week.
4. A week of ketogenic eating with no fasting.
5. A week of very high calorie days. — Remember, we need to balance fasting with feasting.

Whatever you decide, just keep your body on its toes and plan ahead, so it's easy to fit into the schedule and enjoy the extra time!

Why Should I Work Out Then?

I hate to state the truth here, but while working out is still highly recommended, working out isn't going to make a big impact on your weight loss efforts. It's painful for many to comprehend, as it took them so much discipline to get into the groove of working out that it almost feels unnatural not too. There are tons of other benefits of working out aside from weight management.

Health benefits of working out

1. Improved brain health: Regular physical activity can enhance cognitive function and reduce short-term feelings of anxiety.(127)
2. Weight management: Exercise helps prevent excess weight gain and maintain weight loss by burning calories. (128)
3. Reduced risk of diseases: Physical activity can lower the risk of heart diseases, type 2 diabetes, stroke, and some cancers.(129)

4. Strengthened bones and muscles: Exercise helps maintain and improve muscle and bone health. (130)
5. Enhanced mood and mental health: Exercise releases chemicals that can improve mood, self-esteem, and reduce the risk of stress, clinical depression, dementia, and Alzheimer's disease. (127)
6. Increased energy levels: Regular physical activity can boost energy levels and overall productivity. (130)
7. Better sleep quality: Exercise promotes quality sleep and helps fight depression. (127)
8. Delayed signs of aging: Physical activity may delay aging by minimizing bodily inflammation and promoting healthy skin.(131)
9. Improved functional health: Exercise enhances the ability to perform everyday activities and maintain independence as you age. (130)

So we need to shift our mindset as to why we are working out. Resistance training and adding lean muscle is the highest priority, and we will discuss this shortly.

During your long fasts, working out should be kept to walking. Technically, you can do your higher intensity stuff on day one of the fast as you will still have the carbs in your liver and muscles, but you can save that sort of thing for months into the program after you become much more metabolically flexible. Save your weight lifting and other high intensity stuff for 24 hours after the fast is over.

Benefits of adding muscle mass

Now let's talk about muscle mass and its importance in maintaining weight in the future. Adding lean muscle tissue plays a significant role in sustainable weight loss for several reasons. First, lean muscle tissue has a higher metabolic rate compared to fat tissue. By increasing your lean muscle mass, you can enhance your basal metabolic rate (BMR), which is the number of calories your body burns at rest. A higher BMR helps you burn more calories throughout the day, making it harder for you to gain body fat in the future when you are maintaining. (132)

Adding muscle mass also plays a big role in how you look after losing weight. It creates that more firm and tone look most of us desire. The term "skinny fat person" comes to mind. As harsh as that term may sound, it's a common one that refers to the person who lost weight but lost a considerable amount of muscle mass in the process. They feel better about the way they look in clothes, but it's a different story when the clothes start to come off.

Muscle mass will help with the loose skin somewhat. I won't BS you and tell you that it will prevent loose skin, but it can help. Many factors play a role in loose skin development. The biggest being how much weight you lost and your age. I can personally attest that is a big factor in having more unwanted loose skin is the constant yo-yoing that most of you have done in the past. Even though I lost weight at the ripe age of 16, my skin never tightened up fully because I yo-yoed for about a decade afterward. I watched people who lost more than 100 lbs in their 20s and tighten up much more. There is likely a genetic component as well. I reference my 20 plus years in the weight loss space and observing this phenomenon across the board. A side note but cool to mention. I do believe that fasting will tighten skin. I haven't seen any literature that has looked at this. But when you think about the mechanisms at play we discussed regarding cellular autophagy, your body is looking to break down "non-essential" tissues to recycle those proteins for essential tissues. Loose skin seems pretty non-essential to me. I have noticed this to be true when weight loss was done with a more fasting-based approach.

We spoke about workouts and the health benefits. There appears to be some strong evidence suggesting the greater overall benefits is with building and maintaining muscle mass. Several studies have shown that muscle mass is associated with all-cause mortality. In the Nagahama study, skeletal muscle mass index (SMI) was found to be independently associated with all-cause mortality in men.(133) Another study found that reduction in appendicular skeletal muscle mass index (ASMI) was independently associated with a higher mortality rate in patients with heart failure. (134) Furthermore, a study from the CRONICAS cohort found a strong correlation and agreement between skeletal muscle mass (SMM) estimates obtained by the Lee equation and bio-impedance analysis (BIA), with an association between SMM and all-cause mortality existing only when the Lee equation was used. (133) A population-based cohort study in China found that low muscle mass, grip strength, and arm muscle quality were all associated with an increased risk of all-cause mortality. (135) Another study on patients with acute heart failure found that a lower body mass index (BMI) was associated with a higher risk of mortality, and low muscle index (total muscle mass/height^2) was associated with a higher mortality risk. (136)

Save what you got

So how do we reap all these wonderful benefits? The most intelligent way would be to realize you likely have a lot of muscle mass on your frame already, being that you are overweight. This isn't always the case, but either way, you need to protect what you do have. You need to protect the muscle mass that you have on your frame currently. Muscle mass loss is inevitable with weight loss in most cases. You can get into some physique recomposition and focus on both at the same time, but that's more for when you are getting into the athletic body fat ranges. When you can't see your abs as a man or muscle definition in your arms as a woman, then it's best to focus on fat loss as the primary goal. This is what we do with our patients and clients who coach with us beyond their initial fat loss goals. Optimizing hormones and keeping tighter control over more variables is necessary for that. You don't need to worry about that right now. Currently, I want you focused on easy rapid fat loss. I also want you focused on maintaining as much muscle mass as possible throughout your journey!

How do we accomplish this? You already understand from earlier how much the FLOA protocol of fasting significantly optimizes your hormonal profile in favor of muscle mass. But we must produce the signal externally. The signal needs to communicate to the body that your extra skeletal muscle mass is "essential tissue." You will hear me say this over and over; the body is a supercomputer, far exceeding the intelligence of current artificial intelligence in many categories. Not all the categories, of course, just the ones that matter most. 😄 Your body innately knows not to break down organ tissue during fasting or weight loss, or it would die. This is why it would literally be the last tissue to go in a late-stage starvation situation. And even then, it would still choose an intelligent path to organ breakdown, extending survival as far as it possibly can! Truly genius. But extra skeletal muscle isn't innately essential beyond the amount needed to walk around. But if you lift heavy sh** consistently, that changes things around. (137)

So you must adopt a solid resistance training program above all other workouts. In the most time restricted scenarios; as little as two 45-minute workouts can make a significant impact on preserving your lean muscle tissue during your weight loss journey.

170

Ideally, you can commit to 3 weight training sessions per week. And you want to avoid lifting during your long fasting days as well as the day afterward. So that's a 4-day stretch to get 3 weight training sessions in. If you do not have confidence around the gym, then I recommend finding a personal trainer for at least 5 to 10 sessions. You are looking to make a small investment of $200 to $800 here. Emphasize that you are keen to learn a variety of exercises for your major muscle groups and how to work around any injuries that you may have. Furthermore, you desire to learn what real muscle building intensity feels like. After you become comfortable navigating through the gym and performing a high intensity lifting session on your own, then you really don't need a trainer anymore. If you can afford a regular trainer, then, certainly nothing beats a good workout from a trainer, but it falls lower on my totem pole at this point. Make it obvious what your goals are with the trainer. They have the pressure of needing to sell you more sessions. But if you are upfront about not wanting to buy more than the current package for now, it makes things smoother.

This becomes even more relevant when taking one of the GLP-1 medications. There is clear evidence that demonstrates greater muscle mass loss with the use of these medications. It's not the medication causing this. It's the weight loss. Specifically, the daily caloric restriction overtime. These medications are powerful and just get people into greater caloric deficits over time. Hence, the greater initial weight loss and greater rebound weight gained we have discussed. But the beautiful synergy of hormonal optimization produced by the FLOA fasting and our strategy towards calorie cycling really helps to minimize this effect.

High intensity Interval training (HIIT)

After weight training, the next best workout style would be HIIT. But the exact type of HIIT is important to understand. Think "I'm running from a tiger." 3–5 rounds of 20–30 seconds of 100% maximal intensity, followed by 3–4 minutes of rest. That's it! While the total number of calories expended during the workout may be lower than 45 minutes of the stairmaster or elliptical machine; the benefits in the long term are far superior. Using some wisdom here, just look at the body types of sprinters and explosive athletes compared to long-distance runners.

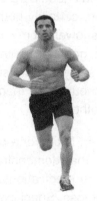
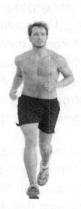

The main reason for this difference is, well, what do you know.... It's an optimization of your hormones again. Are you noticing a trend here yet? Some of these benefits are:

1. Cortisol: HIIT workouts can elevate cortisol levels, which is a stress hormone that aids in the release of fat, especially abdominal and visceral fat. Yes, cortisol can be good when not chronically elevated. (138)
2. Human Growth Hormone (HGH): HIIT has been found to be effective in boosting HGH response, especially in women.

Women have a higher release of HGH in response to intense exercise than men, likely due to higher estrogen levels. HGH helps in burning fat, building muscle, and creating a lean, athletic physique. (139)

3. Testosterone: A single HIIT session can lead to a significant increase in testosterone levels immediately after the workout, but these levels return to baseline values within an hour. Testosterone is an anabolic hormone that helps in muscle growth and recovery. (139)

How to Look at Fasting From a Fresh Perspective

"Fasting rewards you with increased energy. Each time you fast, you will make your mind stronger, and more positive. You will eliminate fear and worry... Fasting helps you to a higher life. Fasting elevates the soul, the mind, and body... By fasting, you can create the person you have always longed to be." — Unknown

The majority of what this quote says can now be scientifically backed. Like anything in life, the barrier of entry exists. Fasting can be challenging for some in the beginning. We must blast through this barrier to be successful. I promise you that it will get easier and easier the more and more you do it. I have provided you with many aids to help you on your journey. I have tried them all myself and I work with our medical practitioners who prescribe the medications to our patients. I have seen first hand what they can do. Get as much help as you can get your hands on, please. This is your health, this is your life, and you only get one. I also gave you some framework to approach the development of a better mindset. Let's apply that towards fasting now.

Mind over matter or mind over hunger

The concept of "mind over matter" refers to the ability to use one's mental strength and willpower to overcome physical limitations or challenges. It suggests that a person can control events, physical objects, or their body's condition using their mind. In essence, it emphasizes the power of the mind to control and influence the body and the physical world in general.(1) How is this possible? Some religions and philosophies believe that you are not your body, but you are the thing that controls your body. I believe this and have experienced it to be true for myself as well. I'm not here to discuss religion or philosophy, I'm here to help you treat your obesity without long-term use of obesity medications.

The thing about religion and philosophy is that we become less scientific, and that can be a problem for many. But I have already pointed out how inaccurate solid sounding science can be at times, so all I'm saying is to try not to be so close minded. Let's play a game here, or better yet; let's run an experiment. I want you to pretend for the next 6 months that you are the thing that indeed runs your body, and you tell it what to do, not the other way around. With this mindset, you make the acknowledgement that you will be starting my FLOA protocol and that you will likely be hungry and tired at many points throughout. But you intend to push through these barriers because it's your decision; despite what feedback your body will give you during those moments. Remind yourself of that big WHY you established earlier. This is the driving force behind many things for you, I presume; not just your weight loss.

Let's understand an important fact about hunger. It's not going to kill you. You cannot die from hunger. You cannot die from a craving being denied. I can throw 100 people on an island with water and salt for 3 weeks plus, even lean athletes, and no one is going to die. In fact, some pretty amazing things would happen to your health on the other end. The longest fast was of a man, Angus

Barbieri, a Scottish man, lasting 382 days from June 1965 to July 1966. At the beginning of his fast, Barbieri weighed 456 pounds (207 kg) and aimed to reach his desired weight of 180 pounds (82 kg). By the end of the fast, he had lost 276 pounds (125 kg) and achieved his weight loss goal. Barbieri was under medical supervision throughout the fast, with doctors conducting regular blood and urine tests to ensure his health was not compromised. After completing his 382-day fast, Angus Barbieri was able to maintain his new weight. Five years after the fast, he weighed 196 pounds (89 kg). (140)

Of course, there may be medical conditions, like diabetes, that would certainly be an exception, but these are rarer than you would think. Many look at the case of Angus like it's so difficult to comprehend, and how in the world could he have done that? Look at the design of the human body. It literally has a storage tank of fuel to keep us alive for that very thing that he did; survive without consuming calories to replenish the storage. The real question you should be asking yourself is:

If we have clinically observed the successful treatment of obesity with the sole intervention of long fasting, why haven't we followed up on this study?

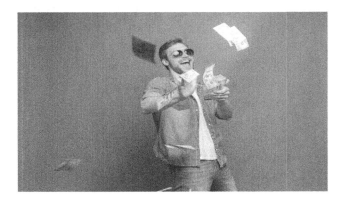

The big pharmaceutical and food industry will do everything it can to suppress treatment options that decrease the need for more medications. History has shown this over and over again. On a positive note, fasting research has made tremendous progress in a general sense and continues to be accepted. It's just sad that it's taken this long to barely progress to where it's currently at.

Dopamine and motivation

We spoke earlier about what long fasting does for mood enhancement. One of my favorite effects is on levels of motivation. Motivation is primarily driven by your brain chemical (neurotransmitter) Dopamine. Other ways to optimize dopamine to improve motivation is constant goal setting and goal attainment. Do you see that beautiful synergy yet? Every time you do a long fast, it's a goal you are setting off to accomplish. If you aren't looking at it that way yet, then I suggest you start to. This will literally improve your motivation levels and make it easier to stay on track with your goals. Additionally, the act itself of long fasting is also enhancing dopamine pathways. Synergy at its finest, if I do say so myself.

Fasting as a Woman

As you know by now, fasting has a massive impact on your hormones. Men have a daily pattern in the release of their hormones. Meaning, every day it's the same pattern we see. This allows for a much more predictable response. Women, on the other hand, have a monthly cycle; specifically 28 days for most women. This means there is a pattern that takes 28 days to complete; therefore it's shifting and changing on the daily. Because of this, women are much more complex and less predictable in terms of how they respond to fasting throughout the 28-day cycle. For a deeper dive into the complexities of a woman's cycle and how to best fast as a woman, I recommend you read the book by Dr. Mindy Pelz: Fasting Like a Girl.

There is a way to navigate through the complexities of a woman's cycle to prevent potential issues and optimize results. Dr. Mindy Pelz's recommendations can be adapted to the FLOA protocol to ensure that women can safely and effectively fast while maintaining hormonal balance.

Fasting During the Menstrual Cycle or Pre-Menopause years

For women with a regular menstrual cycle, the FLOA protocol can be adjusted according to Dr. Pelz's guidelines:

Day 1-12 (Follicular phase): FLOA fast as desired. This phase is characterized by low hormone levels, making it an ideal time for fasting without negatively impacting hormonal balance

Day 11-14 (Ovulation): Estrogen production is at its peak during this time, so it's best to look at 13-16 hour fast to avoid disrupting hormone levels

Days 15-20 (Post Ovulation/Pre luteal phase): Back to FLOA fasting

Day 21-28 (Luteal phase): Progesterone production is at its peak, and fasting should be avoided to prevent anxiety and hormonal shutdown. Increase carb intake to support progesterone production. If you feel great with stage 1 of fasting, then go for it, but really pay attention to how you feel.

I have been working with women for over a decade. My personal experience with women has been such that it does not require such an extreme lack of longer fasting from days 12 until the end. After more recently learning about Dr. Mindy's work, it really does explain the one-offs and difficulties I did see at times. I find that in the most extreme, women have to follow the laid out guidelines above. But in other cases, they can actually get away with longer fasting windows. I think when you are fasting for more weight loss compared to overall health, that this may be the case. Find the perfect balance for yourself in this stage of your life.

Fasting During Peri-Menopause

For peri-menopausal women with erratic menstrual cycles, Dr. Pelz recommends stopping keto and fasting for at least seven days, followed by an increase in carb intake. Magnesium is important. After feeling more stabilized, you can resume the stages above. Due to the decline in progesterone levels compared to earlier in your life, you are even more likely to experience issues with fasting during the final 10 days of your cycle. So pay attention to how you feel and adjust accordingly. Focus on clean carbs choices from your paleo Mediterranean categories.

Post-Menopausal Women

The FLOA protocol can be followed as is for women after menopause. While women still aren't as hormonally stable as men in this stage, they are significantly more stable than ever before.

In summary, adapting the FLOA protocol to a woman's menstrual cycle and life stage is crucial for optimizing hormonal balance and overall health If issues arise.

Understanding how cortisol affects you as a woman

As you learned earlier, cortisol is released during times of stress. The act of fasting is itself a stress, which is why women need to be more careful during their progesterone phase. We also talked about reducing stress to reduce cortisol levels as an overall strategy to aid weight loss. But women should also be even more conscious of their overall stress levels during this stage, as the cortisol will prevent the production of the much-needed progesterone during this stage.

Are there any dangers or concerns here?

"The human body is a miracle of nature, with innate intelligence that allows it to respond to challenges, heal itself, and adapt to survive. It is a testament to the power of life and the resilience of the human spirit." — Unknown

I get asked all the time why I didn't become a medical doctor? With my personal weight struggles, to becoming a personal trainer and then managing trainers; I developed an appreciation for holistic approaches at a very young age. Additionally, I learned from my parents. While they were not in medical themselves, they both arrived at the same conclusion; you need to take responsibility for your health before letting it get to the point where you need medication and surgeries. But it's a great intervention to be used respectively when required. The most powerful concept I learned from my Doctorate of Chiropractic is the innate intelligence that exists within the body. I mention this as we talk about the dangers of fasting.

There are no specific studies that directly link deaths to long fasting, there are cases where complications and deaths have been reported in extreme fasting practices. For instance, a study from 1979 reported cardiovascular complications and deaths in individuals who underwent prolonged fasting or fasting modified by liquid protein supplementation. They were on 4 month fasting protocols.(184) This is literally all that I could dig up about deaths from long fasting protocols.

Regarding safety though, the literature on prolonged fasting, specifically around 48 hours per week, is limited. However, some studies have investigated the safety and efficacy of intermittent fasting and prolonged fasting for shorter durations. A study on people with type 1 diabetes found that 36 hours of prolonged fasting did not increase the risk of hypoglycemia. (141) Another study on insulin-treated type 2 diabetes patients showed that intermittent fasting for 3 nonconsecutive days per week over 12 weeks was safe and improved glycemic control while reducing total daily insulin dose and body weight. (142) A trial on healthy volunteers found that intermittent fasting with a 16-hour fasting period per day for three months significantly improved quality of life and did not raise safety concerns. (143) I think most experts agree that the population of greatest concern for complications from fasting like this would be diabetics. And even for diabetics, it appears it can be safe. Nonetheless, the only real, potentially life-threatening complication that could arise is hypoglycemia. So let's understand it better to add another layer of safety for ourselves.

Hypoglycemia

Hypoglycemia is a potential side effect of long fasting and can be dangerous if you are operating a vehicle or doing anything that requires alertness. This is rare in relatively healthy individuals. But if you jump into a long fast with no intermittent fasting experience, you do increase the likelihood of this. A1C is a measure of your last 3 months of blood sugar and quickly gives you an idea of your body's ability to maintain stable blood sugars. As you creep closer to prediabetes, this is your body telling you that its ability to keep lower is failing. And while fasting is great for rehabilitating this function of the body, the higher the A1C, the higher the likelihood of hypoglycemia during the long fasts due to the normal back and forth blood sugar level rhythms that are altered in diabetics during fasting. Symptoms of hypoglycemia below.

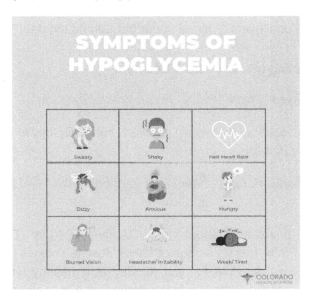

If you have never had a moment of hypoglycemia, then it's likely you won't have this happen, but it's certainly possible. It's good to understand the symptoms, so you can listen to your body if it happens to you. If it happens, then consume some quick acting sugars and call it an end to that fast. Document how long you lasted so that you can beat this fast next time. If this happens, then be sure that you plan your future fasts to be in ideal conditions and not potentially dangerous situations.

This is most likely only going to be a potential issue for diabetics, as their innate blood sugar systems are all jacked up. Diabetics will need less blood sugar lowering medications in a long fast compared to not fasting. A continuous blood glucose monitor would be great, like a dexcom. If you can't get your hands on one, then a standard blood glucose prick and strip method is fine. Check yourself several times a day during your first two weeks of the program on fasting days. Learn the differences in how you feel between eating days and fasting days. Pay attention to how you feel at various levels of blood sugar throughout the day.

Transitioning Into the FLOA Lifestyle

"The first wealth is health." — Ralph Waldo Emerson

"Health is not about the weight you lose, but about the life you gain."
— Unknown (144)

"The groundwork for all happiness is good health." — Leigh Hunt (145)

You have heard a lot about the FLOA lifestyle so far. This is the format of FLOA fasting alongside other lifestyle choices that make it as easy as possible for you to stay at a healthy weight and maintain overall health. It's funny how easy it is to prioritize your health after losing it. First you lose your health, then you lose your quality of life and finally, you lose your life entirely. I'm confident you will find the information in this book valuable. I hope you let it be the vehicle to help you regain your health and quality of life back if you already lost it.

Now that you have returned to a healthy weight, let's keep you there! The golden nugget is this:

Routine rounds of FLOA fasting revolve around intermittent fasting on the other days.

182

This can look like a 48-hour once every 2–4 weeks or a 72-hour once every 3–6 weeks. The body loves variability. A long fast at whatever frequency is maintaining a balance of weight and health for you. To help gauge a balance, I recommend keeping up with the weekly weigh-ins for the rest of your life. While weight and BMI are far from what I would call accurate; it's insanely easy to keep up with. Members of our FLOA lifestyle group enjoy looking back at the last year of weekly weigh-ins and taking a macro look at the graph to isolate what was going on in their lives when they're starting to gain more weight. We have a cool software for them that allows them to do this, and we coach on various strategies to help stay in shape. Skin fold calipers can be very accurate if performed by the same person who has proper training on use. The bioelectrical impedance method is the one you will see the most often due to convenience, but I find it to be very inaccurate at times, which is why it's hard to rely on it. The real accurate measurements of body analysis are:

Dual-Energy X-ray Absorptiometry (DXA Dexa): Dexa scans use X-ray technology to measure bone density, lean tissue mass, and fat mass, providing a comprehensive assessment of body composition (146).

Hydrostatic (Underwater) Weighing: This method involves submerging a person underwater and measuring their weight. The difference between their weight on land and underwater is used to calculate body fat percentage (147).

If you are lucky enough to have access to a facility with hydrostatic weighing or a Dexa scan machine, then I recommend some sort of frequency that you can and are comfortable committing to; such as every 1–6 months. Having objective information allows you to have better control over your health, and your health now depends on maintaining your weight. The funny thing is that you will soon see how much easier your weight will be maintained by keeping insulin levels in check. But I still recommend accountability nonetheless. Furthermore, it's very rewarding to see the results. If you did lose weight in the past, you probably were always let down and constantly frustrated with the weight always seemed to creep Its way back despite your high level of effort to thwart it.

After keeping your fasting schedule in, the rest of it comes down to other effective strategies for keeping your insulin levels lowered, as well as inflammation. Remember, it's all about your hormones more than anything else. The FLOA protocol optimizes your hormones more than any other program period. The exception being actual hormone replacement therapy; in which there is a time and place for. So here are some of the best practices for maintaining overall health and overall hormonal health:

To maintain overall hormonal health, specifically focusing on insulin and leptin, you can follow these best practices:

1. Maintain a balanced diet: Consume a diet rich in whole foods, including a mix of fatty and lean proteins, healthy fats, and complex unrefined carbs. Include lots of color in your produce choices. Avoid processed foods, refined sugars, and unhealthy trans fats.
2. Exercise regularly: Engage in regular physical activity to help regulate insulin and leptin levels. The best form is weight training and proper HIIT.
3. Manage stress: Chronic stress can negatively impact hormonal balance, including insulin and leptin levels. Practice stress-reduction techniques such as mindfulness, meditation, yoga, or deep breathing exercises to help manage stress. (148)

4. Get enough sleep: Aim for 7-9 hours of quality sleep each night. Poor sleep can disrupt hormonal balance, including insulin and leptin levels (148.)
5. Monitor and maintain a healthy weight: Obesity can contribute to insulin resistance and hormonal imbalances. Work towards achieving and maintaining a healthy weight. (149)

Keep a healthy relationship with food. The majority of us are addicted to crappy food. Millions of people who appear to still be very healthy, even with a holistic lens (aka much higher standard of health), are eating crappy food. It's only a matter of time if they continue to consume a diet full of processed crap that it eventually catches up with them. We learned about the strong genetic component that exists for obesity. All this really means is how much harder certain people will have to work at it. This is why I stress the importance of a balanced approach. I advocate for a 90/10 during your program. If you desire to let that fall to an 80/20 then you certainly earned the right to do so. I will argue for this all day, as 80/20 is a hell of a lot better than 50/50! I love the influencers who go to the extreme with their recommendations of a carnivore diet or a 100% whole raw diet. Kudos to them for showing us the potential of what lies within us all to get super serious with our health. It goes back to that entire mind over matter. Oh, and money. The lifestyle that some of these people portray is unattainable because either it's too expensive or requires too much time, which can also be brought back to money, since the majority of us work a 9 to 5 and have kids and all sorts of responsibilities. Find a balance between it all that works for you!

Now what?

Now you can go kick ass in life by accomplishing the very thing that drove you to read this book and drove you to put in the effort all the times you have in the past. Trust me when I say I know how difficult this is, having lived through it myself. This is why I provide multiple levels of support to help you along your journey.

FLOA University

FLOA university is an online course I created on teachable. The course is designed to help you through the implementation of the FLOA protocol. In addition to taking a much deeper dive into various topics discussed within this book; we also cover hundreds of other topics that may come up. Because we also provide live group coaching, it allows us to ensure we are covering every single topic imaginable that every possible person could run into. The course is a lifetime product and I will continue to constantly update it as the latest research presents itself. More importantly, since we actively coach thousands of people across the world, we get to truly see what is working and what isn't, so we can only provide you with the most time effective intel.

The university is organized in a format that makes it very streamlined to follow. You can go through the most important info that everyone needs to and work your way down into all the particulars. It also contains all the theory behind the FLOA protocol as well.

Join our program of live coaching and support

We offer two programs that both consist of live coaching that are designed to personalize and customize your program for the highest level of success. We start off with a live Zoom call that is kept to a small group. As you can imagine, there is a ton of information, so we separated out exactly what you need to know to get started and then this Zoom call is so that we can customize any part of the program for you. After the initial zoom, you are provided access to the private group of members to access the   coaching calls. You get to submit your desired questions and topics a week before each training, and the agenda is posted the day before. Each training is recorded and easily accessible. You are given lifetime access to FLOA university. If you are on a tight schedule, it is posted within the university and broken into its individual topics, so you will be able to access exactly what you desire to access. It's a tremendous group with a live ongoing chat thread and an active community. We also provide a dedicated FLOA hotline, so you can text any personal questions over. Here is my favorite perk:

We provide a guarantee of results.

If you don't lose at least 1% of your body weight per week in either of our live programs, we will continue to coach you at no additional cost until we get you there. I provide this guarantee because I know how frustrating it is to be sold another program and to have all of them tell you this will be the final solution. So rather than try to articulate my confidence, I let the guarantee do it for us.

FLOA Warrior

This is our premier program utilizing the strongest support that science has to provide us yet. We use the combination of Tirzepatide and AOD-9604 to make FLOA fasting as easy as possible. Other peptide/medications combinations exist as well. We perform a comprehensive functional thyroid blood panel and also include pancreatic enzymes to be extra certain the GLP-1 medications won't cause any issues. If need be, we can also optimize your thyroid with bioidentical thyroid hormone. After your blood results, you will have a call with our prescribers to establish the best plan of attack! Currently, we can service most states within the US.

FLOA Practitioner

This is our more economical program. We will utilize some key supplement protocols to aid in your support. The coaching is what really drives this program, and it's very affordable considering that it's done in a group setting. We are open to coaching anyone throughout the globe. The schedule is not an issue because every week you get to post your desired topics and also get the agenda posted beforehand. You still get FLOA hotline access if you struggle with anything. Remember, we guarantee results in this program as well. So if we need to jump on a personal zoom to fix a plateau, It's part of what we do! What people seem to love the most is knowing that if they need the help to keep losing weight, that we are there to move them along.

FLOA Lifestyle

This is the community of people across the world that have lost weight through the FLOA protocol or some fasting-based methods. This group is all about maintaining your health and weight management by implementing the latest and greatest strategies that the literature produces. I also participate in live training 1–2 times per month to support the group. Everyone gets to submit desired topics, and the topics of greater interest will be discussed. What I love most about this group the most is the community that we have developed. There is no other group like this anywhere!

I'm ready to make some serious changes, not only to address my weight, but to improve my overall health. What should I do now?

Obviously, our FLOA™ coaching programs allows us to meet the patients where they are at, and take them from A-Z. The university through is a still a great, start. Don't miss out on this opportunity to transform your health and unlock your full potential.

PLEASE SCAN THE QR CODE TO LEARN MORE ABOUT OUR VARIOUS PROGRAMS:

Appendix

Common Roadblocks and How to Handle Them

The following are common things that can have a big impact on your success. So let's dive in.

High levels of stress

You already learned about cortisol's effect on insulin. High levels of chronic stress can derail your success with the FLOA protocol due to the constant release of cortisol.

It's important to understand that there is such a thing as good stress and to understand the difference between good and bad stress. Good stress, also known as eustress, is a type of stress that can have positive effects on an individual. It can motivate, improve focus, enhance performance, and contribute to personal growth. Examples of good stress include preparing for a presentation, participating in a sports competition, or starting a new job. These situations can be challenging, but ultimately lead to personal growth and satisfaction

On the other hand, bad stress, or distress, is a type of stress that can negatively impact an individual's mental and physical health. It can lead to anxiety, depression, sleep problems, and other health issues. Examples of bad stress include chronic work-related stress, financial stress, or dealing with a traumatic event

The key difference between good and bad stress lies in the way an individual perceives and responds to the stressor. Good stress is typically associated with a sense of challenge and excitement, while bad stress is often linked to feelings of overwhelm, helplessness, and a lack of control. It is important to recognize and manage stress effectively to maintain overall well-being and prevent negative health outcomes

Knowing if you have high-stress levels can be determined by observing various physical, emotional, and behavioral symptoms. Some common indicators of high stress include:

1. Emotional symptoms: Anxiety, irritability, mood swings, feelings of being overwhelmed, and difficulty concentrating (150).
2. Physical symptoms: Muscle tension, headaches, fatigue, sleep disturbances, and changes in appetite (151).
3. Behavioral symptoms: Changes in social interactions, increased use of substances (e.g., alcohol, tobacco, or drugs), and changes in work performance (185)

There are so many ways to handle stress, and the best approach is to find a single or combination of solutions that works for you. Some of the best strategies for managing stress include:

1. Regular exercise: Physical activity can help reduce stress by releasing endorphins, which are natural mood elevators. Exercise also improves overall health and well-being.(152)
2. Slow diaphragmatic breathing: This technique involves taking slow, deep breaths that start from the diaphragm or abdominal area, focusing on abdominal, lung, and chest expansion during the inhale, and a slow, gradual, full release of air on the exhalation. Slow diaphragmatic breathing has been shown to improve psychological and physiological stress responses. (153)
3. Mindfulness meditation: Practicing mindfulness meditation can help you become more aware of your thoughts and feelings, allowing you to better manage stress and anxiety.

(154) Nowadays, you can find so many apps for your phone. Try a few to see which one works best for you.

4. Yoga: Yoga combines physical postures, breathing techniques, and meditation to help reduce stress and anxiety. It has been shown to be effective in managing stress-related health conditions (155).

5. Time management: Prioritizing tasks, setting realistic goals, and breaking tasks into smaller steps can help reduce stress by making your workload more manageable.(156)

6. Social support: Connecting with friends, family, and colleagues can provide emotional support and help you cope with stress (152).

7. Relaxation techniques: Engaging in activities such as listening to music, reading, or taking a warm bath can help you relax and reduce stress (157).

8. Sleep: Ensuring you get enough quality sleep is essential for managing stress, as sleep deprivation can exacerbate stress and anxiety (152). Furthermore, lack of sleep is such a huge common source of stress itself that we will talk about improving sleep shortly.

9. Professional help: If stress becomes overwhelming, consider seeking the help of a mental health professional, such as a therapist or counselor, to help you develop effective stress management strategies (152).

Remember, it's essential to find the stress management techniques that work best for you and incorporate them into your daily routine to effectively manage stress and maintain overall well-being. Testing cortisol levels can be challenging and expensive, so I find it unnecessary most of the time. Using the symptoms above and paying attention to improvements can indicate reduction of perceived stressors and lowered cortisol levels.

Poor sleep

Poor sleep can be defined as having difficulty falling asleep, staying asleep, or experiencing non-restorative sleep, which can lead to daytime dysfunction and reduced quality of life. The literature shows that adult humans require 7 hours of quality sleep each night for optimal response overall.

Poor sleep can lead to alterations in cortisol levels and its daily pattern. For example, children with short sleep duration ($\leq$7.7 hours) displayed higher cortisol awakening response and nadir, while those with low sleep efficiency ($\leq$77.4%) showed higher cortisol levels across the entire day and higher cortisol levels after a stressor (158). In a study on high school students, those with depressive moods and sleep disturbances showed a significant increase in cortisol at 7 am (wake-up time) (159).

Furthermore, poor sleep has been associated with elevated cortisol levels in adults (160). In a study on adolescents and young adults, sleep disturbance was linked to cortisol levels, with stronger effects observed in girls than boys (160). Sleep problems in adolescents have also been linked to hyper-reactivity to stress (160).

Improving the quality of sleep can be achieved through various strategies, including:

1. Maintain a consistent sleep schedule: Going to bed and waking up at the same time every day helps regulate your body's internal clock, making it easier to fall asleep and wake up refreshed (161).
2. Turn out the lights an hour before bed. If you need some light, get a red bulb.
3. Drop the temperature to 65-68 F. If your partner hates it, then invest in a cooling machine for your side of the bed.

4. Avoid caffeine intake after 12-2pm. Caffeine has a ½ life of 5 to 6 hours. Even if you can fall asleep with caffeine consumed later, as I can, it has been shown to reduce the quality of your sleep.
5. Create a sleep-friendly environment: Ensure your bedroom is cool, dark, and quiet. Use blackout curtains, earplugs, or white noise machines to block out disturbances (162).
6. Limit EMF Exposure. EMF stands for electromagnetic fields that are emitted from various electronic devices. The biggest culprits are cell phones that are looking for signals and Wi-Fi devices. Put your phone on airplane mode before bed, and find a better spot in the house than your bedroom for the Wi-Fi router.
7. Limit exposure to screens before bedtime: The blue light emitted by phones, tablets, and computers can interfere with your sleep. Try to avoid using these devices at least an hour before bed (162).
8. Practice relaxation techniques: Engaging in activities such as deep breathing, meditation, or progressive muscle relaxation can help calm your mind and prepare your body for sleep (163).
9. Stop eating 3–4 hours before bedtime.
10. Exercise regularly: Regular physical activity can help you fall asleep faster and enjoy deeper sleep. However, avoid intense workouts close to bedtime, as they may have the opposite effect (164).

Low thyroid hormones

If you are unable to get a complete functional thyroid panel, and you suspect low thyroid symptoms, then I strongly recommend you find a clinic like ours that can check for you and medicate if necessary. Make sure they use a desiccated thyroid like Armor Thyroid or Natures Thyroid.

If you want to get your thyroid levels checked by us then please reach out by scanning the QR Code.

Excessive inflammation

Excessive inflammation can be caused by various factors, including tissue damage, infections, and immune system dysregulation. Some of the main causes of excessive inflammation include:

1. Diet diet diet – A diet full of processed foods will drive a ton of inflammation.
2. Autoimmune diseases – Autoimmune diseases involve the dysregulation of the immune system, leading to an exaggerated immune response that causes tissue damage and inflammation. Inflammatory cytokines play a significant

195

FAST, FEAST, & FLOURISH

role in the development and progression of these diseases (165).

3. Tissue damage: Damaged and dying cells release molecules called damage-associated molecular patterns (DAMPs), which promote sterile inflammation. This type of inflammation is important for tissue repair and regeneration but can also lead to the development of numerous inflammatory diseases, such as metabolic disorders, neurodegenerative diseases, autoimmune diseases, and cancer (166).

4. Infections: Inflammatory responses can be triggered by bacterial, viral, or fungal infections.(167)

5. Inflammatory pathways: Activation of certain molecular pathways, can drive inflammation in various disease settings, including infection, cellular stress, and tissue damage (168).

6. Chronic inflammatory diseases: Conditions like chronic inflammatory bowel disease can trigger excessive inflammation in other parts of the body. For example, gut inflammation has been shown to activate certain signaling, initiating the formation of processes in the brain and contributing to Alzheimer's disease (169)

The following are effective strategies to help lower inflammation:

Adopt an anti-inflammatory diet: Focus on consuming foods rich in dietary fiber, probiotics, antioxidants, and omega-3 fatty acids, while reducing the intake of red meat, processed meat, and added sugar (170).

1. Follow an autoimmune diet: The same idea of an anti-inflammatory diet but even more restrictive. Things like gluten and other triggers must be avoided as they produce strong inflammation within the body.

2. The combination of curcumin and resveratrol has been shown to have synergistic anti-inflammatory effects. (171). Dietary supplementation of combined curcumin (500mg/kg) and resveratrol (200mg/kg) also synergistically reduce vascular inflammation in mice (171). The combination of curcumin and resveratrol protects against vascular inflammation by suppressing signaling in both in vitro and in vivo models (171).

3. Exercise regularly: Engaging in regular physical activity can help reduce inflammation by promoting an anti-inflammatory phenotype in the general population (172). Exercise intensity and duration can be adjusted to suit individual needs and preferences.

4. Practice healthy emotion regulation strategies: Emotion regulation strategies like reappraisal have been associated with lower levels of inflammation, while maladaptive strategies like suppression have been linked to higher inflammation levels (173). Developing healthy emotion regulation skills can help mitigate the effects of stress on inflammation.

5. Maintain a healthy weight: Obesity is a known risk factor for chronic inflammation. Achieving and maintaining a healthy weight through a balanced diet and regular exercise can help reduce inflammation levels.

6. Manage stress: Chronic stress can contribute to inflammation. Incorporating stress management techniques, such as mindfulness meditation, yoga, or deep breathing exercises, can help reduce stress and its impact on inflammation.

7. Get enough sleep: Poor sleep quality and sleep deprivation have been linked to increased inflammation. Aim for 7-9 hours of quality sleep per night to support overall health and reduce inflammation.

Alcohol

Alcohol is a topic that often comes up in discussions about weight loss and overall health. It's important to understand its effects on the body, particularly when following the FLOA protocol

Physical Health Impacts

Alcohol can have a significant impact on weight loss efforts. It's high in calories, can stimulate the appetite, and typically leads to poor food choices. Furthermore, alcohol can negatively affect metabolic processes, impairing the body's ability to burn fat. It can also contribute to other health issues such as liver disease, cardiovascular problems, and certain types of cancer

In the context of the FLOA protocol, drinking alcohol near your long fasting windows can disrupt the fasting process in many ways. Alcohol will dehydrate you, so it will increase the chances of becoming dehydrated during your fast. Moreover, you will likely deal with abnormal patterns of hunger during your fast as your body continues to detoxify, thus making it more challenging to complete your fast. Finally, alcohol is a major disruptor of quality sleep. Just because you are actually asleep does not mean it's quality sleep. A lot of the fasting benefits happen when you sleep! Therefore, it's recommended to avoid alcohol around your fasting windows. We shouldn't sugar coat it here:

There are no physical benefits to drinking alcohol, only harm to our health.

Mental Health Considerations

While the physical health impacts of alcohol are generally negative, it's important to consider its role in social situations and mental

198

health. For some, moderate alcohol consumption can serve as a social lubricant, helping to reduce anxiety and facilitate social interactions. This can contribute to improved mental health and overall well-being.

Alcohol and the FLOA Protocol: A Balanced Approach

Given the potential negative impacts of alcohol on physical health and its potential role in social situations and mental health, a balanced approach is recommended when following the FLOA protocol. During your weight loss journey and while restoring optimal health with the FLOA protocol, it's advisable to reduce or eliminate alcohol consumption. This will help to maximize the benefits of the protocol and support your weight loss efforts

Once you've achieved your weight loss goals and restored your health, you may choose to reintroduce alcohol in moderation, if you feel it contributes positively to your social interactions or mental well-being. However, it's important to treat alcohol like "cheat food" – to be used sparingly and consciously. Meaning, you should set yourself up with some parameters or rules to follow. It's nice to eb and flow with life, but where has that gotten you so far? Create some policies for yourself and stick to it.

A fresh perspective on alcohol

While I do consider the effects of alcohol to aid in social interaction, which is absolutely essential to a human's mental health, it is crucial to remember that alcohol is not a necessary component for socializing or mental health. There are many other ways to manage stress and foster social connections that do not involve alcohol. You should do your best to have a good time without the need to drink. Test the waters for yourself and just do it once: refrain from drinking in a social setting where you would normally otherwise. Let's pick an appropriate occasion first, if you have different events where you drink to different degrees. Let's start with the lightest settings, where you have 1 – 2 drinks, for example. Take note of how you feel during the event. Was it really all that bad? Was the only thing that really affected you what you thought others may think? Here is one of many golden rules I live by:

Nobody really gives a sh** what you do or don't do. Most pretend to care, but really only if it serves their needs.

Work your way after this point. Maybe where you drink a heavier amount, try drinking less and see what happens. You may be surprised how different the world actually is depending on how much you drink! LOL. But in all fairness, how much of a difference was it reducing your 5 glasses of wine to 2 or 3?

Remember, the goal is not to ban alcohol completely, but to understand its impacts on your health and make informed decisions about its place in your lifestyle. As with all aspects of the FLOA protocol, the key is balance and sustainability.

Examples of various starting points

Obese Woman with a weight of 250lbs and Pre-Diabetes that is non medicated

Jane is a 45-year-old woman who weighs 250 lbs and has pre-diabetes. She has never fasted before. She started the FLOA protocol with the goal of losing weight, but she was also afraid of becoming a diabetic. Furthermore, she had the understanding that addressing her insulin resistance was a key factor in her pre-diabetes condition. Despite the more common approach of working their way into the deeper FLOA fasting stages from stage one, Jane decided to jump in head first. During our initial coaching call, I explained how both scenarios looked, and It made much more sense to her to approach it this rapid way. Our medical practitioners prescribed her Tirzepatide and AOD-9604 to help her out with the massive hunger and energy issues we expected her to experience.

In the first week, Jane begins with a 36-hour fast, consuming only water and coffee during the fast. She was only able to accomplish a 24 on her, first go around. She did use the Unimate and Calocurb as well during long fasts. She was capable of hitting the 36-hour fast on her 3rd attempt. She described the first long fasts as very challenging, but was determined to see them through. There were points during her first fasts where she wanted to eat her desk, as she would describe, but she kept herself distracted as much as possible with work and various activities. She broke her fasts with bone broth first and then later would consume other soups with chicken and vegetables

Over the following weeks, Jane gradually increases the duration of her fasts to 48 hours. She is always ensuring she is well-hydrated and monitoring her blood sugar levels. After a few weeks of noticing how stable her blood sugar was, she stopped checking. She noticed improvements in her energy levels. After 3 months on the FLOA protocol, Jane has lost 40 lbs, and her blood sugar levels have stabilized. After another 8 months following the FLOA protocol, she reached her target weight of 150lbs. She really emphasized the variability of her weekly FLOA fasting, ensuring she switched it up every month or so.

She continues with the FLOA lifestyle, incorporating less frequent rounds of fasting and maintaining a healthy diet

Example 2: Woman with a weight of 190 and Some Experience in Intermittent Fasting

Sarah is a 35-year-old woman who weighs 190 lbs and has tried intermittent fasting in the past but struggled with consistency. She has no official medical conditions yet, but she admits to feeling like crap with low levels of energy and lots of abdominal fat. She decides to try the FLOA protocol to achieve more sustainable results

Sarah starts the FLOA protocol on her own. She purchased the online course and felt very determined. After completing the course and attending some group trainings that come along with it, Sarah was ready to begin. She approached it very slowly and methodically. She started with stage one fasting for an 8-hour eating window for 3 weeks. After this became easy, she then progressed to adding a 24-hour fast once per week. After a few weeks, she added two. She felt like the Unimate and Calocurb were really helping her make the fast easier, as she had never fasted this much and managed to stay consistent. Finally, 3 months into it, she started with the FLOA fasting stage. First with a 36 and then working closer to the goal of 48 which she hit by month 4.

She finds that the structure of the FLOA protocol helps her maintain consistency, and she enjoys the freedom of eating more on her non-fasting days. After 8 months, Sarah hit her goal weight of 140lbs. She feels more energetic and healthier. She continues with the FLOA lifestyle, incorporating less frequent rounds of fasting and maintaining a balanced diet. She added HIIT training to her regime 2-3x week after her weight training sessions. She only works out 3 times per week but is very consistent. Furthermore, she finds it's so much less stressful not feeling guilty about wanting and feeling like she needed to go 6 times a week but unable to with her busy work and family life.

Anti-Inflammatory Diets

Autoimmune protocol

This is an example of a more extreme restrictive diet approach. If you have an autoimmune disease or think you are inflamed, it's a must. By implementing the dietary strategies discussed in this book, you are already reducing inflammation, but some of you will need this more extreme approach. The idea is to go very strict for 3 months and then start to re-introduce some foods back in one at a time, one week at a time. You need to fully assess any changes in symptoms and avoid anything that causes a negative reaction. Build on your list of foods that were well tolerated.

Foods to avoid

1. Grains: rice, wheat, oats, barley, rye, etc., as well as foods derived from them, such as pasta, bread, and breakfast cereal
2. Legumes: lentils, beans, peas, peanuts, etc., as well as foods derived from them, such as tofu, tempeh, mock meats, or peanut butter
3. Nightshade vegetables: eggplants, peppers, potatoes, tomatoes, tomatillos, etc., as well as spices derived from nightshade vegetables, such as paprika
4. Eggs: whole eggs, egg whites, or foods containing these ingredients
5. Dairy: cow's, goat's, or sheep's milk, as well as foods derived from these milks, such as cream, cheese, butter, or ghee; dairy-based protein powders or other supplements should also be avoided
6. Nuts and seeds: all nuts and seeds and foods derived from them, such as flours, butter, or oils; also includes cocoa and

seed-based spices, such as coriander, cumin, anise, fennel, fenugreek, mustard, and nutmeg
7. Certain beverages: alcohol and coffee
8. Processed vegetable oils: canola, rapeseed, corn, cottonseed, palm kernel, safflower, soybean, or sunflower oils
9. Refined or processed sugars: cane or beet sugar, corn syrup, brown rice syrup, and barley malt syrup; also includes sweets, soda, candy, frozen desserts, and chocolate, which may contain these ingredients
10. Food additives and artificial sweeteners: trans fats, food colorings, emulsifiers, and thickeners, as well as artificial sweeteners, such as stevia, mannitol, and xylitol

Foods to eat

1. Vegetables: various vegetables except for nightshade vegetables and algae, which should be avoided
2. Fresh fruit: various fresh fruit, in moderation
3. Tubers: sweet potatoes, taro, yams, as well as Jerusalem or Chinese artichokes
4. Minimally processed meat: wild game, fish, seafood, organ meat, and poultry; meats should be wild, grass-fed or pasture-raised, whenever possible
5. Fermented, probiotic-rich foods: nondairy-based fermented food, such as kombucha, sauerkraut, pickles, and coconut kefir; probiotic supplements may also be consumed
6. Minimally processed vegetable oils: olive oil, avocado oil, or coconut oil
7. Herbs and spices: as long as they're not derived from a seed or a chili pepper
8. Vinegars: balsamic, apple cider, and red wine vinegar, as long as they're free of added sugars

9. Certain teas: green and black tea at average intakes of up to 3–4 cups per day
10. Bone broth

OMAD aka One Meal a Day

I get asked about OMAD a lot due to my love and appreciation for the longer style of fasting. The OMAD (One Meal a Day) diet is a form of intermittent fasting that involves fasting for 23 hours and consuming one large meal within a 60-minute window. From a perspective of accomplishing the hormonal changes that we need to, OMAD is very powerful at accomplishing this. The problem with OMAD that I have noticed with patients and myself is the difficulty of eating enough. It is challenging to get in enough calories, protein, fiber and micro nutrients when you are eating only once per day. This is why we opt for 2–3 meals outside your FLOA fasting days. You can still benefit from OMAD by using it occasionally, as this is perfectly fine. This is what stage one of fasting really is; two OMADs in the week. Once you are in the FLOA lifestyle, you can throw in some OMADs intentionally. Just stay away from doing it more than 3 days in a row on any consistency basis.

High Intensity Interval Training Done right

High-Intensity Interval Training (HIIT) is a popular form of exercise that combines short bursts of intense activity with periods of rest or lower-intensity exercise. There are various forms of HIIT out there. It has become an umbrella term for any form of exercise that falls into this category of altering intensities. Because of this, it is difficult to generalize the benefits. Of all the possible ways of performing alterations, I truly believe the best style is the one called the "One Minute Workout." This program was developed by Martin Gibala and Christopher Shulgan, as detailed in their book of the same name. What makes this form unique is that it is the most intense form of HIIT that one can perform.

In the fitness arena, we refer to the difficulty of an exercise as the Rating of Perceived Exertion (RPE). It's a subjective measure used to quantify the intensity of physical activity based on an individual's perception of their exertion during exercise. Most programs do not even speak of an RPE, but some do. With the ones that do, they usually advocate an RPE somewhere between 50-75/80% of the max during the harder interval and somewhere between 0-40 for the lighter period. In The One Minute Workout, we are going as close to 100% excretion as possible. This is where the name came from because each round focuses on 20-second bursts of as close to 100% RPE as one can go. Think "I'm running from a tiger." This is followed by 3–4 minutes of rest. The idea being that if you didn't need the full 3–4 minutes of rest, then you didn't go hard enough. This is considered one round, and you only need to complete 3-5 rounds for the workout. Be sure to perform a good warm-up and cooldown

The benefits of the "One Minute Workout" are backed by research, which has shown that short bursts of high-intensity exercise can be as effective as longer, moderate-intensity workouts for improving health and fitness.(174) HIIT has been studied in sedentary adults and people with various health conditions, such as heart failure and Type 2 diabetes (175) (176) (177). The main reason why this form of HIIT far exceeds other forms is the greater degree of hormonal optimization that results. If you paid attention to this book, you understand that this is why FLOA is so magical. The body generally responds to stressors proportionally to the degree of the stressor itself.

In these cases, "smarter" happens to also be harder. ☺

References

A. Wilding JPH, Batterham RL, Davies M, et al. Weight regain and cardiometabolic effects after withdrawal of semaglutide: The STEP 1 trial extension. Diabetes Obes Metab. 2022;24(8):1553-1564. doi:10.1111/dom.14725

1. Steinbeck, Kate S. "The future of obesity management." *Clinical obstetrics and gynecology* vol. 47,4 (2004): 942-56; discussion 980-1. doi:10.1097/01.grf.0000135418.61892.d9

2. Whitley, Andrea, and Najat Yahia. "Efficacy of Clinic-Based Telehealth vs. Face-to-Face Interventions for Obesity Treatment in Children and Adolescents in the United States and Canada: A Systematic Review." *Childhood obesity (Print)* vol. 17,5 (2021): 299-310. doi:10.1089/chi.2020.0347

3. Whitley, Andrea, and Najat Yahia. "Efficacy of Clinic-Based Telehealth vs. Face-to-Face Interventions for Obesity Treatment in Children and Adolescents in the United States and Canada: A Systematic Review." *Childhood obesity (Print)* vol. 17,5 (2021): 299-310. doi:10.1089/chi.2020.0347

4. Flegal, Katherine M et al. "Association of all-cause mortality with overweight and obesity using standard body mass index categories: a systematic review and meta-analysis." *JAMA* vol. 309,1 (2013): 71-82. doi:10.1001/jama.2012.113905

5. Köchli, Sabrina et al. "Obesity, High Blood Pressure, and Physical Activity Determine Vascular Phenotype in Young Children." *Hypertension (Dallas, Tex. : 1979)* vol. 73,1 (2019): 153-161. doi:10.1161/HYPERTENSIONAHA.118.11872

6. Danaei, Goodarz. "Abstract SY02-03: Mediators of the effect of overweight and obesity on cardiovascular disease and cancer: Evidence from pooling of prospective studies." *Cancer Research* 75 (2015): n. pag.

7. Cao, Li et al. "Effects of Body Mass Index, Waist Circumference, Waist-to-Height Ratio and Their Changes on Risks of Dyslipidemia among Chinese Adults: The Guizhou Population Health Cohort Study." *International journal of environmental research and public health* vol. 19,1 341. 29 Dec. 2021, doi:10.3390/ijerph19010341

8. Chew, Han Shi Jocelyn et al. "Sustainability of Weight Loss Through Smartphone Apps: Systematic Review and Meta-analysis on Anthropometric, Metabolic, and Dietary Outcomes." *Journal of medical Internet research* vol. 24,9 e40141. 21 Sep. 2022, doi:10.2196/40141

9. Stefanaki, Katerina et al. "Obesity and hyperandrogenism are implicated with anxiety, depression and food cravings in women with polycystic ovary syndrome." *Endocrine* vol. 82,1 (2023): 201-208. doi:10.1007/s12020-023-03436-1

10. Chaturvedi, Shakti et al. "Stigma and Discrimination: the Twain Impact on Mental Health During COVID-19 Pandemic." *Trends in Psychology*, 1–20. 13 Apr. 2022, doi:10.1007/s43076-022-00179-2

11. Ryal, Joed Jacinto et al. "Effects of a Multi-Professional Intervention on Mental Health of Middle-Aged Overweight Survivors of COVID-19: A Clinical Trial." *International journal of environmental research and public health* vol. 20,5 4132. 25 Feb. 2023, doi:10.3390/ijerph20054132

12. Armenta-Hernández, Oziely Daniela et al. "Impact of job strain and being overweight on middle and senior managers from the manufacturing sector in the Mexican industry." *Work (Reading, Mass.)* vol. 69,3 (2021): 1027-1040. doi:10.3233/WOR-213533

13. Lazzeroni, Matteo et al. "A Meta-Analysis of Obesity and Risk of Colorectal Cancer in Patients with Lynch Syndrome: The Impact of Sex and Genetics." *Nutrients* vol. 13,5 1736. 20 May. 2021, doi:10.3390/nu13051736

14. Ogden, Cynthia L. Ph.D., and Margaret D. Carroll, M.S.P.H., Division of Health and Nutrition Examination Surveys. "Prevalence of Overweight, Obesity, and Extreme Obesity Among Adults: United States Trends 1960–1962 Through 2007–2008"

15. Tai, M M et al. "Meal size and frequency: effect on the thermic effect of food." *The American journal of clinical nutrition* vol. 54,5 (1991): 783-7. doi:10.1093/ajcn/54.5.783

16. Pes, Giovanni Mario et al. "Evolution of the Dietary Patterns Across Nutrition Transition in the Sardinian Longevity Blue Zone and Association with Health Indicators in the Oldest Old." *Nutrients* vol. 13,5 1495. 28 Apr. 2021, doi:10.3390/nu13051495

17. Hales, Craig M et al. "Prevalence of Obesity and Severe Obesity Among Adults: United States, 2017-2018." *NCHS data brief* ,360 (2020): 1-8.

18. Wang, Youfa et al. "Has the prevalence of overweight, obesity and central obesity levelled off in the United States? Trends, patterns, disparities, and future projections for the obesity epidemic." *International journal of epidemiology* vol. 49,3 (2020): 810-823. doi:10.1093/ije/dyz273

19. He, Yuan et al. "Prevalence of Underweight, Overweight, and Obesity Among Reproductive-Age Women and Adolescent Girls in Rural China." *American journal of public health* vol. 106,12 (2016): 2103-2110. doi:10.2105/AJPH.2016.303499

20. Lawler, Katherine et al. "Leptin-Mediated Changes in the Human Metabolome." *The Journal of clinical endocrinology*

and metabolism vol. 105,8 (2020): 2541–2552. doi:10.1210/clinem/dgaa251

21. Tan, Bowen et al. "Cellular and molecular basis of leptin resistance." *bioRxiv* (2023): n. Pag.

22. Machairiotis, Nikolaos et al. "Inflammatory Mediators and Pain in Endometriosis: A Systematic Review." *Biomedicines* vol. 9,1 54. 8 Jan. 2021, doi:10.3390/biomedicines9010054

23. Jastrząb, Anna et al. "Cannabidiol Regulates the Expression of Keratinocyte Proteins Involved in the Inflammation Process through Transcriptional Regulation." *Cells* vol. 8,8 827. 3 Aug. 2019, doi:10.3390/cells8080827

24. Sun, Lizhong et al. "Fibroblast membrane-camouflaged nanoparticles for inflammation treatment in the early stage." *International journal of oral science* vol. 13,1 39. 16 Nov. 2021, doi:10.1038/s41368-021-00144-2

25. Schulte, Fabian et al. "The relationship between specialized pro-resolving lipid mediators, morbid obesity and weight loss after bariatric surgery." *Scientific reports* vol. 10,1 20128. 18 Nov. 2020, doi:10.1038/s41598-020-75353-6

26. Jiang, Zhihui et al. "Protective Effects of 1,8-Cineole Microcapsules Against Inflammation and Gut Microbiota Imbalance Associated Weight Loss Induced by Heat Stress in Broiler Chicken." *Frontiers in pharmacology* vol. 11 585945. 14 Jan. 2021, doi:10.3389/fphar.2020.585945

27. Del Chierico, Federica et al. "The impact of intestinal microbiota on weight loss in Parkinson's disease patients: a pilot study." *Future microbiology* vol. 15 (2020): 1393-1404. doi:10.2217/fmb-2019-0336

28. Bahceci, M et al. "The correlation between adiposity and adiponectin, tumor necrosis factor alpha, interleukin-6 and high sensitivity C-reactive protein levels. Is adipocyte size associated with inflammation in adults?." *Journal of*

endocrinological investigation vol. 30,3 (2007): 210-4. doi:10.1007/BF03347427

29. Tangvarasittichai, Surapon et al. "Tumor Necrosis Factor-A, Interleukin-6, C-Reactive Protein Levels and Insulin Resistance Associated with Type 2 Diabetes in Abdominal Obesity Women." *Indian journal of clinical biochemistry : IJCB* vol. 31,1 (2016): 68-74. doi:10.1007/s12291-015-0514-0

30. Hummasti, Sarah, and Gökhan S Hotamisligil. "Endoplasmic reticulum stress and inflammation in obesity and diabetes." *Circulation research* vol. 107,5 (2010): 579-91. doi:10.1161/CIRCRESAHA.110.225698

31. Meiliana, Anna and Andi Yasmin Wijaya. "Metaflammation, NLRP3 Inflammasome Obesity and Metabolic Disease." *The Indonesian Biomedical Journal* 3 (2011): 168.

32. Conger, Krista. "Can you repeat that? The crisis in research reliability". Stanford Medicine. 15 Aug. 2016, (https://stanmed.stanford.edu/can-you-repeat-that/)

33. Gautam, Monica. "Evolution Of Food Culture Through Timeline." *International Journal of Research* 5 (2018): 193-197.

34. Simons, E L. "Human origins." *Science (New York, N.Y.)* vol. 245,4924 (1989): 1343-50. doi:10.1126/science.2506640

35. Yuan, Xiaojie et al. "Effect of Intermittent Fasting Diet on Glucose and Lipid Metabolism and Insulin Resistance in Patients with Impaired Glucose and Lipid Metabolism: A Systematic Review and Meta-Analysis." *International journal of endocrinology* vol. 2022 6999907. 24 Mar. 2022, doi:10.1155/2022/6999907

36. Yun, Hyung-Mun et al. "Xanol Promotes Apoptosis and Autophagy and Inhibits Necroptosis and Metastasis via the Inhibition of AKT Signaling in Human Oral Squamous Cell

Carcinoma." *Cells* vol. 12,13 1768. 3 Jul. 2023, doi:10.3390/cells12131768

37. Zhao, Qiang et al. "Naringenin Exerts Cardiovascular Protective Effect in a Palmitate-Induced Human Umbilical Vein Endothelial Cell Injury Model via Autophagy Flux Improvement." *Molecular nutrition & food research* vol. 63,24 (2019): e1900601. doi:10.1002/mnfr.201900601

38. Yue, Chaoxiong et al. "Autophagy Is a Defense Mechanism Inhibiting Invasion and Inflammation During High-Virulent *Haemophilus parasuis* Infection in PK-15 Cells." *Frontiers in cellular and infection microbiology* vol. 9 93. 16 Apr. 2019, doi:10.3389/fcimb.2019.00093

39. Van Dyck, Lisa et al. "OR16-4 The Growth Hormone Axis in Relation to Muscle Weakness in the ICU: Effect of Early Macronutrient Deficit." *Journal of the Endocrine Society* vol. 3,Suppl 1 OR16-4. 30 Apr. 2019, doi:10.1210/js.2019-OR16-4

40. Tian, Miao. "Effect of Exogenous Growth Hormone on Growth and Skeletal Muscle Hyperplasia and Hypertrophy of Nile Tilapia(Oreochromis niloticus)." *Journal of Agriculture Biotechnology* (2012): n. Pag.

41. Matsukawa, Shino et al. "Activation of the β-adrenergic receptor exacerbates lipopolysaccharide-induced wasting of skeletal muscle cells by increasing interleukin-6 production." *PloS one* vol. 16,5 e0251921. 18 May. 2021, doi:10.1371/journal.pone.0251921

42. Thomsen, Henrik H et al. "Effects of 3-hydroxybutyrate and free fatty acids on muscle protein kinetics and signaling during LPS-induced inflammation in humans: anticatabolic impact of ketone bodies." *The American journal of clinical nutrition* vol. 108,4 (2018): 857-867. doi:10.1093/ajcn/nqy170

43. Wijngaarden, Marjolein A et al. "Effects of prolonged fasting on AMPK signaling, gene expression, and mitochondrial respiratory chain content in skeletal muscle from lean and obese individuals." *American journal of physiology. Endocrinology and metabolism* vol. 304,9 (2013): E1012-21. doi:10.1152/ajpendo.00008.2013

44. Ezpeleta, Mark et al. "Efficacy and safety of prolonged water fasting: a narrative review of human trials." *Nutrition reviews*, nuad081. 27 Jun. 2023, doi:10.1093/nutrit/nuad081

45. Decker, Kevin. "Nutritional strategies for the exercise-induced increases in brain-derived neurotrophic factor." *The Journal of physiology* vol. 601,11 (2023): 2217-2218. doi:10.1113/JP284482

46. Doney, Ellen et al. "Inflammation-driven brain and gut barrier dysfunction in stress and mood disorders." *The European journal of neuroscience* vol. 55,9-10 (2022): 2851-2894. doi:10.1111/ejn.15239

47. Wallace, C W et al. "Effect of fasting on dopamine neurotransmission in subregions of the nucleus accumbens in male and female mice." *Nutritional neuroscience* vol. 25,7 (2022): 1338-1349. doi:10.1080/1028415X.2020.1853419

48. Bastani, Abdolhossein et al. "The Effects of Fasting During Ramadan on the Concentration of Serotonin, Dopamine, Brain-Derived Neurotrophic Factor and Nerve Growth Factor." *Neurology international* vol. 9,2 7043. 23 Jun. 2017, doi:10.4081/ni.2017.7043

49. Stringer, Eleah et al. "Intermittent Fasting in Cancer: a Role in Survivorship?." *Current nutrition reports* vol. 11,3 (2022): 500-507. doi:10.1007/s13668-022-00425-0

50. Salvadori, Giulia et al. "Intermittent and Periodic Fasting, Hormones, and Cancer Prevention." *Cancers* vol. 13,18 4587. 13 Sep. 2021, doi:10.3390/cancers13184587

51. Kim, Joo Hyun et al. "CXCR4 can induce PI3Kδ inhibitor resistance in ABC DLBCL." *Blood cancer journal* vol. 8,2 23. 22 Feb. 2018, doi:10.1038/s41408-018-0056-9

52. Nakashima, Kazuki, and Aiko Ishida. "Regulation of Autophagy in Chick Skeletal Muscle: Effect of mTOR Inhibition." *The journal of poultry science* vol. 57,1 (2020): 77-83. doi:10.2141/jpsa.0190008

53. Tinsley, Grant M, and Benjamin D Horne. "Intermittent fasting and cardiovascular disease: current evidence and unresolved questions." *Future cardiology* vol. 14,1 (2018): 47-54. doi:10.2217/fca-2017-0038

54. Mohamed, Ahmed Ismail et al. "Ramadan Intermittent Fasting and Its Beneficial Effects of Health: A Review Article." (2020).

55. Tavernarakis, Nektarios. "Regulation and Roles of Autophagy in the Brain." *Advances in experimental medicine and biology* vol. 1195 (2020): 33. doi:10.1007/978-3-030-32633-3_5

56. Gudden, Jip et al. "The Effects of Intermittent Fasting on Brain and Cognitive Function." *Nutrients* vol. 13,9 3166. 10 Sep. 2021, doi:10.3390/nu13093166

57. Włodarek, Dariusz. "Role of Ketogenic Diets in Neurodegenerative Diseases (Alzheimer's Disease and Parkinson's Disease)." *Nutrients* vol. 11,1 169. 15 Jan. 2019, doi:10.3390/nu11010169

58. Tavernarakis, Nektarios. "Regulation and Roles of Autophagy in the Brain." *Advances in experimental medicine and biology* vol. 1195 (2020): 33. doi:10.1007/978-3-030-32633-3_5

59. Morales-Suarez-Varela, María et al. "Intermittent Fasting and the Possible Benefits in Obesity, Diabetes, and Multiple Sclerosis: A Systematic Review of Randomized Clinical

Trials." *Nutrients* vol. 13,9 3179. 13 Sep. 2021, doi:10.3390/nu13093179

60. Shimokawa, I, and Y Higami. "Leptin and anti-aging action of caloric restriction." *The journal of nutrition, health & aging* vol. 5,1 (2001): 43-8.

61. Hoshino, Shunsuke et al. "Mechanisms of the anti-aging and prolongevity effects of caloric restriction: evidence from studies of genetically modified animals." *Aging* vol. 10,9 (2018): 2243-2251. doi:10.18632/aging.101557

62. Longo, Valter D et al. "Intermittent and periodic fasting, longevity and disease." *Nature aging* vol. 1,1 (2021): 47-59. doi:10.1038/s43587-020-00013-3

63. McCarthy, Cameron G. et al. "β-Hydroxybutyrate (βOHB) Activates Gpr109a to Contribute to the Anti-vascular Aging Effect of Autophagy." *The FASEB Journal* 34 (2020): n. Pag.

64. Yamamuro, Tadashi et al. "Loss of RUBCN/rubicon in adipocytes mediates the upregulation of autophagy to promote the fasting response." *Autophagy* vol. 18,11 (2022): 2686-2696. doi:10.1080/15548627.2022.2047341

65. Joaquim, Lisandra et al. "Benefits, mechanisms, and risks of intermittent fasting in metabolic syndrome and type 2 diabetes." *Journal of physiology and biochemistry* vol. 78,2 (2022): 295-305. doi:10.1007/s13105-021-00839-4

66. Ucci, Sarassunta et al. "Thyroid Hormone Protects from Fasting-Induced Skeletal Muscle Atrophy by Promoting Metabolic Adaptation." *International journal of molecular sciences* vol. 20,22 5754. 15 Nov. 2019, doi:10.3390/ijms20225754

67. Tao, Xiao-Li et al. "The effects of autophagy on the replication of Nelson Bay orthoreovirus." *Virology journal* vol. 16,1 90. 18 Jul. 2019, doi:10.1186/s12985-019-1196-7

68. Wang, Youli et al. "Impact of Different Durations of Fasting on Intestinal Autophagy and Serum Metabolome in Broiler

Chicken." *Animals : an open access journal from MDPI* vol. 11,8 2183. 23 Jul. 2021, doi:10.3390/ani11082183

69. Berger, Bettina et al. "Seven-day fasting as a multimodal complex intervention for adults with type 1 diabetes: Feasibility, benefit and safety in a controlled pilot study." *Nutrition (Burbank, Los Angeles County, Calif.)* vol. 86 (2021): 111169. doi:10.1016/j.nut.2021.111169

70. Thakur, Milind et al. "A HOSPITAL BASED PROSPECTIVE STUDY TO COMPARE THE EFFICACY AND SAFETY OF ROPIVACAINE FENTANYL AND BUPIVACAINE FENTANYL USING INTRATHECAL IN LOWER LIMB ORTHOPEDIC SURGERIES." (2023).

71. He, Yuying et al. "The clinical effect and safety of new preoperative fasting time guidelines for elective surgery: a systematic review and meta-analysis." *Gland surgery* vol. 11,3 (2022): 563-575. doi:10.21037/gs-22-49

72. Shiju, Rashmi et al. "Safety Assessment of Glucose-Lowering Drugs and Importance of Structured Education during Ramadan: A Systematic Review and Meta-Analysis." *Journal of diabetes research* vol. 2022 3846253. 18 Feb. 2022, doi:10.1155/2022/3846253

73. Bello, Nicholas T, and Matthew R Zahner. "Tesofensine, a monoamine reuptake inhibitor for the treatment of obesity." *Current opinion in investigational drugs (London, England : 2000)* vol. 10,10 (2009): 1105-16.

74. Szczepańska, Ewa, and Małgorzata Gietka-Czernel. "FGF21: A Novel Regulator of Glucose and Lipid Metabolism and Whole-Body Energy Balance." *Hormone and metabolic research = Hormon- und Stoffwechselforschung = Hormones et metabolisme* vol. 54,4 (2022): 203-211. doi:10.1055/a-1778-4159

75. Stinson, Stephen. "UNCERTAIN CLIMATE FOR ANTIHISTAMINES: Side effects that caused FDA to move

against Seldane also occur with at least one other nonsedating antihistamine." *Chemical & Engineering News* 75 (1997): 43-45.

76. Psaty, Bruce M et al. "A lifecycle approach to the evaluation of FDA approval methods and regulatory actions: opportunities provided by a new IOM report." *JAMA* vol. 307,23 (2012): 2491-2. doi:10.1001/jama.2012.5545

77. Davidson, Michael H. "Rosuvastatin safety: lessons from the FDA review and post-approval surveillance." *Expert opinion on drug safety* vol. 3,6 (2004): 547-57. doi:10.1517/14740338.3.6.547

78. Vandenplas, Y, and ESPGHAN Cisapride Panel. European Society for Pediatric Gastroenterology, Hepatology and Nutrition. "Current pediatric indications for cisapride." *Journal of pediatric gastroenterology and nutrition* vol. 31,5 (2000): 480-9. doi:10.1097/00005176-200011000-00006

79. Vandenplas, Y, and ESPGHAN Cisapride Panel. European Society for Pediatric Gastroenterology, Hepatology and Nutrition. "Current pediatric indications for cisapride." *Journal of pediatric gastroenterology and nutrition* vol. 31,5 (2000): 480-9. doi:10.1097/00005176-200011000-00006

80. Tucker, G T et al. "Optimizing drug development: strategies to assess drug metabolism/transporter interaction potential--towards a consensus." *British journal of clinical pharmacology* vol. 52,1 (2001): 107-17. doi:10.1046/j.0306-5251.2001.temp.1441.x

81. Svorcan, Petar et al. "The influence of intraabdominal pressure on the mortality rate of patients with acute pancreatitis." *Turkish journal of medical sciences* vol. 47,3 748-753. 12 Jun. 2017, doi:10.3906/sag-1509-7

82. Wang, Rongzhi et al. "What Lies Beneath? - Medullary Thyroid Cancer in Nodular Graves' Disease." *Journal of the Endocrine Society* 5 (2021): n. Pag.

83. Proch, Jędrzej et al. "Influence of Brewing Method on the Content of Selected Elements in Yerba Mate (*Ilex paraguarensis*) Infusions." *Foods (Basel, Switzerland)* vol. 12,5 1072. 2 Mar. 2023, doi:10.3390/foods12051072

84. Borges, Maria Carolina et al. "The effect of mate tea (Ilex paraguariensis) on metabolic and inflammatory parameters in high-fat diet-fed Wistar rats." *International journal of food sciences and nutrition* vol. 64,5 (2013): 561-9. doi:10.3109/09637486.2012.759188

85. Kang, Young-Rye et al. "Anti-obesity and anti-diabetic effects of Yerba Mate (Ilex paraguariensis) in C57BL/6J mice fed a high-fat diet." *Laboratory animal research* vol. 28,1 (2012): 23-9. doi:10.5625/lar.2012.28.1.23

86. Yimam, Mesfin et al. "Appetite Suppression and Antiobesity Effect of a Botanical Composition Composed of *Morus alba*, *Yerba mate*, and *Magnolia officinalis*." *Journal of obesity* vol. 2016 (2016): 4670818. doi:10.1155/2016/4670818

87. Masson, Walter et al. "Effect of Yerba Mate (Ilex paraguariensis) on Lipid Levels: A Systematic Review and Meta-Analysis." *Plant foods for human nutrition (Dordrecht, Netherlands)* vol. 77,3 (2022): 353-366. doi:10.1007/s11130-022-00991-2

88. Reicks, Marla et al. "Total dietary fiber intakes in the US population are related to whole grain consumption: results from the National Health and Nutrition Examination Survey 2009 to 2010." *Nutrition research (New York, N.Y.)* vol. 34,3 (2014): 226-34. doi:10.1016/j.nutres.2014.01.002

89. Walker, Edward et al. "New Zealand Bitter Hops Extract Reduces Hunger During a 24 h Water Only Fast." *Nutrients* vol. 11,11 2754. 13 Nov. 2019, doi:10.3390/nu11112754

90. "Bitter Orange." *National Center for Complementary Integrative Health*, Updated 1 May 2020, (www.nccih.nih.gov/health/bitter-orange).

91. Chen, H., Vlahos, R., Bozinovski, S. *et al.* Effect of Short-Term Cigarette Smoke Exposure on Body Weight, Appetite and Brain Neuropeptide Y in Mice. *Neuropsychopharmacol* 30, 713–719 (2005). (https://doi.org/10.1038/sj.npp.1300597)

92. Stojakovic, Andrea, Enma P Espinosa, Osman T Farhad, and Kabirullah Lutfy. "Effects of nicotine on homeostatic and hedonic components of food intake". *Journal of Endocrinology* 235.1 (2017): R13-R31. < (https://doi.org/10.1530/JOE-17-0166>). Web. 4 Oct. 2023.

93. Hindmarch, I et al. "Effects of nicotine gum on psychomotor performance in smokers and non-smokers." *Psychopharmacology* vol. 100,4 (1990): 535-41. doi:10.1007/BF02244008

94. Goveia, Elyse. "Just Say "Nootropic": The Effects of Nicotine on Memory and Learning." (2008).

95. Al Asoom, Lubna et al. "The Effectiveness of *Nigella sativa* and Ginger as Appetite Suppressants: An Experimental Study on Healthy Wistar Rats." *Vascular health and risk management* vol. 19 1-11. 10 Jan. 2023, doi:10.2147/VHRM.S396295

96. Stuby, Johann et al. "Appetite-Suppressing and Satiety-Increasing Bioactive Phytochemicals: A Systematic Review." *Nutrients* vol. 11,9 2238. 17 Sep. 2019, doi:10.3390/nu11092238

97. Gupta, Charu et al. "Appetite Suppressing Phyto Nutrients: Potential for Combating Obesity." *Journal of Nutritional Health & Food Engineering* 3 (2015): n. Pag.

98. Rosenbaum, Michael, and Gary Foster. "Differential mechanisms affecting weight loss and weight loss maintenance." *Nature metabolism* vol. 5,8 (2023): 1266-1274. doi:10.1038/s42255-023-00864-1

99. Everitt, Arthur V, and David G Le Couteur. "Life extension by calorie restriction in humans." *Annals of the New York Academy of Sciences* vol. 1114 (2007): 428-33. doi:10.1196/annals.1396.005

100. Dornas, Waleska C et al. "Health implications of high-fructose intake and current research." *Advances in nutrition (Bethesda, Md.)* vol. 6,6 729-37. 13 Nov. 2015, doi:10.3945/an.114.008144

101. Zhang, Wei et al. "TRIB3 mediates glucose-induced insulin resistance via a mechanism that requires the hexosamine biosynthetic pathway." *Diabetes* vol. 62,12 (2013): 4192-200. doi:10.2337/db13-0312

102. Singh, Ram B. et al. "Nutrition in Transition from Homo sapiens to Homo economicus." *The Open Nutraceuticals Journal* 6 (2013): 6-17.

103. Corley, Janie et al. "Dietary factors and biomarkers of systemic inflammation in older people: the Lothian Birth Cohort 1936." *The British journal of nutrition* vol. 114,7 (2015): 1088-98. doi:10.1017/S000711451500210X

104. Tolkien, Katie et al. "An anti-inflammatory diet as a potential intervention for depressive disorders: A systematic review and meta-analysis." *Clinical nutrition (Edinburgh, Scotland)* vol. 38,5 (2019): 2045-2052. doi:10.1016/j.clnu.2018.11.007

105. Romagnolo, Donato F, and Ornella I Selmin. "Mediterranean Diet and Prevention of Chronic Diseases." *Nutrition today* vol. 52,5 (2017): 208-222. doi:10.1097/NT.0000000000000228

106. Silva, Carolina F M et al. "Effect of ultra-processed foods consumption on glycemic control and gestational weight gain in pregnant with pregestational diabetes mellitus using carbohydrate counting." *PeerJ* vol. 9 e10514. 1 Feb. 2021, doi:10.7717/peerj.10514

107.   Cordova, Reynalda et al. "Consumption of ultra-processed foods associated with weight gain and obesity in adults: A multi-national cohort study." *Clinical nutrition (Edinburgh, Scotland)* vol. 40,9 (2021): 5079-5088. doi:10.1016/j.clnu.2021.08.009

108.   Kearns, Cristin E et al. "Sugar Industry and Coronary Heart Disease Research: A Historical Analysis of Internal Industry Documents." *JAMA internal medicine* vol. 176,11 (2016): 1680-1685. doi:10.1001/jamainternmed.2016.5394

109.   Epner, Margeaux et al. "Understanding the Link between Sugar and Cancer: An Examination of the Preclinical and Clinical Evidence." *Cancers* vol. 14,24 6042. 8 Dec. 2022, doi:10.3390/cancers14246042

110.   Cash, Sean B. et al. "Integrating Food Policy with Growing Health and Wellness Concerns: An Analytical Literature Review of the Issues Affecting Government, Industry, and Civil Society." *Project Report Series* (2005): n. Pag.

111.   Gómez, Eduardo J. "Coca-Cola's political and policy influence in Mexico: understanding the role of institutions, interests and divided society." *Health policy and planning* vol. 34,7 (2019): 520-528. doi:10.1093/heapol/czz063

112.   Dhaka, Vandana et al. "Trans fats-sources, health risks and alternative approach - A review." *Journal of food science and technology* vol. 48,5 (2011): 534-41. doi:10.1007/s13197-010-0225-8

113.   Jahromi, Mitra Kazemi et al. "Adherence to diet with higher dietary diabetes risk reduction score is associated with reduced risk of type 2 diabetes incident in Iranian adults." *BMC public health* vol. 23,1 1144. 14 Jun. 2023, doi:10.1186/s12889-023-16024-9

114.   Carpenter, Kelly M et al. "A Randomized Pilot Study of a Phone-Based Mindfulness and Weight Loss Program."

Behavioral medicine (Washington, D.C.) vol. 45,4 (2019): 271-281. doi:10.1080/08964289.2017.1384359

115.   Kwak, Soyoung, and Min Cheol Chang. "Impaired consciousness due to injury of the ascending reticular activating system in a patient with bilateral pontine infarction: A case report." *Translational neuroscience* vol. 11,1 264-268. 24 Aug. 2020, doi:10.1515/tnsci-2020-0138

116.   Abbas, Naaz et al. "Microbial production of docosahexaenoic acid (DHA): biosynthetic pathways, physical parameter optimization, and health benefits." *Archives of microbiology* vol. 205,9 321. 29 Aug. 2023, doi:10.1007/s00203-023-03666-x

117.   Hei, Abdul. "Mental Health Benefits of Fish Consumption." (2021).

118.   Moyad, Mark A. "Osteoporosis. Part III--Not just for bone loss: potential benefits of calcium and vitamin D for overall general health." *Urologic nursing* vol. 23,1 (2003): 69-74.

119.   Palermo, Nadine E, and Michael F Holick. "Vitamin D, bone health, and other health benefits in pediatric patients." *Journal of pediatric rehabilitation medicine* vol. 7,2 (2014): 179-92. doi:10.3233/PRM-140287

120.   Ferrillo, Martina et al. "Oral Health in Breast Cancer Women with Vitamin D Deficiency: A Machine Learning Study." *Journal of clinical medicine* vol. 11,16 4662. 9 Aug. 2022, doi:10.3390/jcm11164662

121.   Peng, Ying et al. "Anti-Inflammatory Effects of Curcumin in the Inflammatory Diseases: Status, Limitations and Countermeasures." *Drug design, development and therapy* vol. 15 4503-4525. 2 Nov. 2021, doi:10.2147/DDDT.S327378

122.   Meng, Xiao et al. "Health Benefits and Molecular Mechanisms of Resveratrol: A Narrative Review." *Foods*

(Basel, Switzerland) vol. 9,3 340. 14 Mar. 2020, doi:10.3390/foods9030340

123.   Kaur, Arshpreet et al. "Resveratrol: A Vital Therapeutic Agent with Multiple Health Benefits." *Drug research* vol. 72,1 (2022): 5-17. doi:10.1055/a-1555-2919

124.   Wallace, Robert G.. "Models of vascular injury and the potential therapeutic benefits of magnesium supplementation." (2020).

125.   Mikalsen, Solveig Meyer et al. "Improved Magnesium Levels in Morbidly Obese Diabetic and Non-diabetic Patients After Modest Weight Loss." *Biological Trace Element Research* 188 (2018): 45 - 51.

126.   Cant find

127.   Hashimoto, Takeshi et al. "Effect of Exercise on Brain Health: The Potential Role of Lactate as a Myokine." *Metabolites* (2021): n. Pag.

128.   Calleja, Melissa et al. "Increased dairy product consumption as part of a diet and exercise weight management program improves body composition in adolescent females with overweight and obesity-A randomized controlled trial." *Pediatric obesity* vol. 15,12 (2020): e12690. doi:10.1111/ijpo.12690

129.   Ballin, Marcel, and Peter Nordström. "Does exercise prevent major non-communicable diseases and premature mortality? A critical review based on results from randomized controlled trials." *Journal of internal medicine* vol. 290,6 (2021): 1112-1129. doi:10.1111/joim.13353

130.   Ahuja, Dr. Anil and Deepti Mathpal. "An Analysis of Health Benefits of Exercise." *International Journal of Innovative Research in Engineering & Management* (2022): n. Pag.

131.   Wu, Ne N et al. "Physical Exercise and Selective Autophagy: Benefit and Risk on Cardiovascular Health."

Cells vol. 8,11 1436. 14 Nov. 2019, doi:10.3390/cells8111436

132.   Marks, B L, and J M Rippe. "The importance of fat free mass maintenance in weight loss programmes." *Sports medicine (Auckland, N.Z.)* vol. 22,5 (1996): 273-81. doi:10.2165/00007256-199622050-00001

133.   Tabara, Yasuharu et al. "Skeletal muscle mass index is independently associated with all-cause mortality in men: The Nagahama study." *Geriatrics & gerontology international* vol. 22,11 (2022): 956-960. doi:10.1111/ggi.14491

134.   Katano, Satoshi et al. "Anthropometric parameters-derived estimation of muscle mass predicts all-cause mortality in heart failure patients." *ESC heart failure* vol. 9,6 (2022): 4358-4365. doi:10.1002/ehf2.14121

135.   Wu, Man et al. "Associations of muscle mass, strength, and quality with all-cause mortality in China: a population-based cohort study." *Chinese medical journal* vol. 135,11 1358-1368. 5 Jun. 2022, doi:10.1097/CM9.0000000000002193

136.   Hwang, In-Chang et al. "Body Mass Index, Muscle Mass, and All-Cause Mortality in Patients With Acute Heart Failure: The Obesity Paradox Revisited." *International journal of heart failure* vol. 4,2 95-109. 4 Apr. 2022, doi:10.36628/ijhf.2022.0007

137.   Butt, Ahmad G.. "The Impact of Resistance Exercise on Skeletal Muscle in Older Adults: A Literature Review." (2021).

138.   Irandoust, Khadijeh and Morteza Taheri. "Effect of a High Intensity Interval Training (HIIT) on Serotonin and Cortisol Levels in Obese Women With Sleep Disorders." *Women's Health Bulletin* (2018): n. Pag.

139. Gharahdaghi, Nima et al. "Links Between Testosterone, Oestrogen, and the Growth Hormone/Insulin-Like Growth Factor Axis and Resistance Exercise Muscle Adaptations." *Frontiers in physiology* vol. 11 621226. 15 Jan. 2021, doi:10.3389/fphys.2020.621226

140. Washburn, Kevin E et al. "Hairy vetch (Vicia villosa) toxicosis in a purebred Angus herd." *The Bovine Practitioner* (2007): n. Pag.

141. Moser, Othmar et al. "712-P: Safety and Efficacy of 36 Hours Prolonged Fasting on Glucose Metabolism in People with Type 1 Diabetes: A Crossover Trial." *Diabetes* 69 (2020): n. Pag.

142. Varady, Krista A et al. "Clinical application of intermittent fasting for weight loss: progress and future directions." *Nature reviews. Endocrinology* vol. 18,5 (2022): 309-321. doi:10.1038/s41574-022-00638-x

143. Saluja, Manoj et al. " Study of Impact of Glycemic Status (HbA1c) on Platelet Activity measured by Mean Platelet Volume & Vascular Complications in Diabetics." *The Journal of the Association of Physicians of India* vol. 67,4 (2019): 26-29.

144. Yasmin, Neha. "60 Health Is Wealth Quotes To Motivate You To Live A Healthier Life." *Vantage Fit*, 4 Mar. 2022, (www.vantagefit.io/blog/health-is-wealth-quotes/).

145. VOGEL, KAITLIN. "In a Health Rut? These 100 Quotes Will Inspire You to Get Back on Track." *Parade*, 18 May 2023, parade.com/1179956/kaitlin-vogel/health-quotes/.

146. Duren, Dana L et al. "Body composition methods: comparisons and interpretation." *Journal of diabetes science and technology* vol. 2,6 (2008): 1139-46. doi:10.1177/193229680800200623

147.	SATRAZEMIS, EMMIE .RD, CSSD . "What Is Body Composition? 5 Ways to Measure Body Fat." *Parade*, 23 Mar. 2021, (www.trifectanutrition.com/blog/what-is-body-composition-and-how-to-measure-it).

148.	Brogan, Kelly et al. "Psychotropic Drug Withdrawal and Holistic Tapering Strategies: A Case Series." *Advances in mind-body medicine* vol. 33,4 (2019): 4-16.

149.	Anand-Ivell, Ravinder et al. "Association of age, hormonal, and lifestyle factors with the Leydig cell biomarker INSL3 in aging men from the European Male Aging Study cohort." *Andrology* vol. 10,7 (2022): 1328-1338. doi:10.1111/andr.13220

150.	Luceño-Moreno, Lourdes et al. "Symptoms of Posttraumatic Stress, Anxiety, Depression, Levels of Resilience and Burnout in Spanish Health Personnel during the COVID-19 Pandemic." *International journal of environmental research and public health* vol. 17,15 5514. 30 Jul. 2020, doi:10.3390/ijerph17155514

151.	Lou, Hu et al. "The impact of adolescents' health motivation on the relationship among mental stress, physical exercise, and stress symptoms during COVID-19: A dual moderation model." *Frontiers in public health* vol. 11 1164184. 11 Apr. 2023, doi:10.3389/fpubh.2023.1164184

152.	Shahzadi, Asifa et al. "Stress Management Strategies Used by Nurses to Regain Energy at Work Place." *Saudi Journal of Nursing and Health Care* (2022): n. Pag.

153.	Bentley, Tanya G K et al. "Slow-Breathing Curriculum for Stress Reduction in High School Students: Lessons Learned From a Feasibility Pilot." *Frontiers in rehabilitation sciences* vol. 3 864079. 1 Jul. 2022, doi:10.3389/fresc.2022.864079

154. Agarwal, Suresh Kumar. "Stress relief techniques based on Patanjali Yoga Sutra." (2013).

155. Gupta, Neetika et al. "YOGA-A Holistic Approach For Stress Management In Dentistry -"Part And Parcel Of Life"." (2021).

156. Ogomegbunam, Odita Anthony. "Stress Management Strategies and Employee Performance: An Application of Correlational Research Design on Manufacturing Firms in Edo State, Nigeria." *JOURNAL OF ECONOMICS, FINANCE AND MANAGEMENT STUDIES* (2023): n. Pag.

157. Mitthun, A. N. K. et al. "Evaluation of Various Stress Management Strategies among Chennai People - A Cross Sectional Study." *Journal of Pharmaceutical Research International* (2021): n. Pag.

158. Räikkönen, Katri et al. "Poor sleep and altered hypothalamic-pituitary-adrenocortical and sympatho-adrenal-medullary system activity in children." *The Journal of clinical endocrinology and metabolism* vol. 95,5 (2010): 2254-61. doi:10.1210/jc.2009-0943

159. Yu, Minjoon et al. "Changes in Hormones, Melatonin and Cortisol, Related to the Psychological and Sleep States of High School Students." *Oral health* 2 (2018): 1-8.

160. Kische, Hanna et al. "ODP029 Associations between Objective and Subjective Indicators of Stress and Sleep Disturbance in Adolescents and Young Adults from the General Population." *Journal of the Endocrine Society* vol. 6,Suppl 1 A54–A55. 1 Nov. 2022, doi:10.1210/jendso/bvac150.112

161. Packer, Sharon. "Sleep Hygiene Tips to Prevent Insomnia." (2020).

162. Knapik, Joseph J et al. "Sleep and Injuries in Military Personnel With Suggestions for Improving Sleep and

Mitigating Effects of Sleep Loss." *Journal of special operations medicine : a peer reviewed journal for SOF medical professionals* vol. 22,4 (2022): 102-110. doi:10.55460/X89P-KV2Q

163.   Packer, Sharon. "Sleep Hygiene Tips to Prevent Insomnia." (2020).

164.   Packer, Sharon. "Sleep Hygiene Tips to Prevent Insomnia." (2020).

165.   Ogbodo, John Onyebuchi et al. "Volatile organic compounds: A proinflammatory activator in autoimmune diseases." *Frontiers in immunology* vol. 13 928379. 29 Jul. 2022, doi:10.3389/fimmu.2022.928379

166.   Gong, Tao et al. "DAMP-sensing receptors in sterile inflammation and inflammatory diseases." *Nature reviews. Immunology* vol. 20,2 (2020): 95-112. doi:10.1038/s41577-019-0215-7

167.   Schauer, Anja E et al. "IL-37 Causes Excessive Inflammation and Tissue Damage in Murine Pneumococcal Pneumonia." *Journal of innate immunity* vol. 9,4 (2017): 403-418. doi:10.1159/000469661

168.   Decout, Alexiane et al. "The cGAS-STING pathway as a therapeutic target in inflammatory diseases." *Nature reviews. Immunology* vol. 21,9 (2021): 548-569. doi:10.1038/s41577-021-00524-z

169.   Chen, Chun et al. "Gut inflammation triggers C/EBPβ/δ-secretase-dependent gut-to-brain propagation of Aβ and Tau fibrils in Alzheimer's disease." *The EMBO journal* vol. 40,17 (2021): e106320. doi:10.15252/embj.2020106320

170.   Keshteli, Ammar Hassanzadeh et al. "Anti-Inflammatory Diet Prevents Subclinical Colonic Inflammation and Alters Metabolomic Profile of Ulcerative

Colitis Patients in Clinical Remission." *Nutrients* vol. 14,16 3294. 11 Aug. 2022, doi:10.3390/nu14163294

171. Zhang, Lijuan et al. "Synergistic anti-inflammatory effects and mechanisms of the combination of resveratrol and curcumin in human vascular endothelial cells and rodent aorta." *The Journal of nutritional biochemistry* vol. 108 (2022): 109083. doi:10.1016/j.jnutbio.2022.109083

172. Metsios, George S et al. "Exercise and inflammation." *Best practice & research. Clinical rheumatology* vol. 34,2 (2020): 101504. doi:10.1016/j.berh.2020.101504

173. Appleton, Allison A et al. "Divergent associations of adaptive and maladaptive emotion regulation strategies with inflammation." *Health psychology : official journal of the Division of Health Psychology, American Psychological Association* vol. 32,7 (2013): 748-56. doi:10.1037/a0030068

174. Gibala, Martin J et al. "Physiological adaptations to low-volume, high-intensity interval training in health and disease." *The Journal of physiology* vol. 590,5 (2012): 1077-84. doi:10.1113/jphysiol.2011.224725

175. Pescatello, Linda S et al. "Exercise for Hypertension: A Prescription Update Integrating Existing Recommendations with Emerging Research." *Current hypertension reports* vol. 17,11 (2015): 87. doi:10.1007/s11906-015-0600-y

176. Boutcher, Stephen H. "High-intensity intermittent exercise and fat loss." *Journal of obesity* vol. 2011 (2011): 868305. doi:10.1155/2011/868305

177. Pattyn, Nele et al. "Aerobic interval training vs. moderate continuous training in coronary artery disease patients: a systematic review and meta-analysis." *Sports medicine (Auckland, N.Z.)* vol. 44,5 (2014): 687-700. doi:10.1007/s40279-014-0158-x

178.   Kottusch, Pia et al. "Oberlebenszeit bei Nahrungs-
und Flüssigkeitskarenz" [Survival time without food and
drink]. *Archiv fur Kriminologie* vol. 224,5-6 (2009): 184-91.
179.   García-Rodríguez, Darío, and Alfredo Giménez-
Cassina. "Ketone Bodies in the Brain Beyond Fuel
Metabolism: From Excitability to Gene Expression and Cell
Signaling." *Frontiers in molecular neuroscience* vol. 14
732120. 27 Aug. 2021, doi:10.3389/fnmol.2021.732120
180.   Decker, Kevin. "Nutritional strategies for the
exercise-induced increases in brain-derived neurotrophic
factor." *The Journal of physiology* vol. 601,11 (2023): 2217-
2218. doi:10.1113/JP284482
181.   Wallace, C W et al. "Effect of fasting on dopamine
neurotransmission in subregions of the nucleus accumbens
in male and female mice." *Nutritional neuroscience* vol. 25,7
(2022): 1338-1349. doi:10.1080/1028415X.2020.1853419
182.   Giannakou, Konstantinos et al. "The effect of
intermittent fasting on cancer prevention: a systematic
review." *European Journal of Public Health* 30 (2020): n.
Pag.
183.   Tavernarakis, Nektarios. "Regulation and Roles of
Autophagy in the Brain." *Advances in experimental
medicine and biology* vol. 1195 (2020): 33. doi:10.1007/978-
3-030-32633-3_5
184.   Isner, J M et al. "Sudden, unexpected death in avid
dieters using the liquid-protein-modified-fast diet.
Observations in 17 patients and the role of the prolonged
QT interval." *Circulation* vol. 60,6 (1979): 1401-12.
doi:10.1161/01.cir.60.6.1401
185.   Luceño-Moreno L, Talavera-Velasco B, García-
Albuerne Y, Martín-García J. Symptoms of Posttraumatic
Stress, Anxiety, Depression, Levels of Resilience and
Burnout in Spanish Health Personnel during the COVID-19

Pandemic. *Int J Environ Res Public Health*. 2020;17(15):5514. Published 2020 Jul 30. doi:10.3390/ijerph17155514

186.   Wilding, John P H et al. "Weight regain and cardiometabolic effects after withdrawal of semaglutide: The STEP 1 trial extension." *Diabetes, obesity & metabolism* vol. 24,8 (2022): 1553-1564. doi:10.1111/dom.14725

12407672R00134